Clinical Analytics and Data Management for the DNP

Martha L. Sylvia, PhD, MBA, RN, is assistant professor at the Johns Hopkins University School of Nursing with a joint appointment in the School of Medicine, and an associate faculty member of the Welch Center for Prevention, Epidemiology, and Clinical Research. She is the director of the Population Health Analytics Core, a unit that is jointly sponsored by Johns Hopkins HealthCare; Johns Hopkins Welch Center for Prevention, Epidemiology, and Clinical Research; and the Division of General Internal Medicine. Dr. Sylvia currently participates in four research projects with Johns Hopkins University, including serving as the principal investigator on Calculating Cost Savings for Care Management Programs (Johns Hopkins HealthCare) and as principal investigator on An Evaluation of The Access Program (TAP) at East Baltimore Medical Center (Johns Hopkins Community Physicians and Urban Health Institute). She has published eight peer-reviewed research papers; has presented internationally on data management and predictive analytics in Australia, Germany, Japan, and Malaysia; and has presented nationally at the American Association of Colleges of Nursing (AACN) Doctoral Conference, America's Health Insurance Plans (AHIP), and the American Society of Health Risk Management, among many others. Dr. Sylvia developed and has taught 3 years of both sections I and II of the Clinical Data Management course in the Doctor of Nursing Practice (DNP) program at Johns Hopkins. She has over 10 years experience in clinical analytics and 10 years clinical nursing experience in acute care medical–surgical nursing, provider office staff nursing, case management, management of community and health plan case management services, and executive leadership of a community-based free clinic for the uninsured.

Mary F. Terhaar, DNSc, RN, is associate professor at the Johns Hopkins University School of Nursing and director of the Doctor of Nursing Practice program. Dr. Terhaar is currently principal investigator on several projects sponsored by the Maryland Health Services Cost Review Commission, including "Needs-Based Graduate Education" and "Stimulating Practice Innovation." She is also co-investigator on the "Guiding Initiative for Doctoral Education" and the "Faculty Leadership Development Institute." All studies focus on increasing the number of doctorally prepared nurses and promoting quality care and nursing education. She has published extensively in peer-reviewed journals; has presented internationally on collaborative practice, outcomes management, performance improvement in education, and DNP education and practice in Hong Kong, Russia, Canada, Taiwan, Australia, and Switzerland; and has presented nationally at the AACN Doctoral Education Conference, and many others. Dr. Terhaar evaluated the scholarly work products from early DNP graduates and identified the need to increase the quality and rigor of the translation activities and project evaluations.

Clinical Analytics and Data Management for the DNP

Martha L. Sylvia, PhD, MBA, RN

Mary F. Terhaar, DNSc, RN

SPRINGER PUBLISHING COMPANY

NEW YORK

Springer Publishing Company, LLC
11 West 42nd Street
New York, NY 10036
www.springerpub.com

Acquisitions Editor: Margaret Zuccarini
Composition: Amnet Systems

ISBN: 978-0-8261-2973-4
e-book ISBN: 978-0-8261-2974-1

17 / 6

The author and the publisher of this Work have made every effort to use sources believed to be reliable to provide information that is accurate and compatible with the standards generally accepted at the time of publication. Because medical science is continually advancing, our knowledge base continues to expand. Therefore, as new information becomes available, changes in procedures become necessary. We recommend that the reader always consult current research and specific institutional policies before performing any clinical procedure. The author and publisher shall not be liable for any special, consequential, or exemplary damages resulting, in whole or in part, from the readers' use of, or reliance on, the information contained in this book. The publisher has no responsibility for the persistence or accuracy of URLs for external or third-party Internet websites referred to in this publication and does not guarantee that any content on such websites is, or will remain, accurate or appropriate.

Library of Congress Cataloging-in-Publication Data

Sylvia, Martha L., author.
  Clinical analytics and data management for the DNP / Martha L. Sylvia,
Mary F. Terhaar.
    p. ; cm.
  Includes bibliographical references and index.
  ISBN 978-0-8261-2973-4 (print) — ISBN 978-0-8261-2974-1 (e-book)
  I. Terhaar, Mary F., author. II. Title.
  [DNLM: 1. Advanced Practice Nursing—education. 2. Nursing Research—methods.
3. Data Collection—methods. 4. Data Interpretation, Statistical. WY 18.5]
  RT81.5
  610.73072—dc23
                                                                          2013051313

Printed in the United States of America by Bradford & Bigelow.

This book is dedicated to Amy, an admirable nurse and lovely niece.

Contents

Contributors

Shannon Murphy, MA
Biostatistician
Care Management Department, Outcomes and Research Unit
Johns Hopkins HealthCare LLC, Baltimore, MD

Melissa Sherry, MPH, CPH
Research Associate
Johns Hopkins HealthCare LLC, Baltimore, MD

Foreword

Clinical Analytics and Data Management for the DNP is a most welcome addition to the available resources for nurses in advanced practice and executive roles. The book is unique. It aims to provide nurses with the analytic skills needed to transform practice at the systems level, and thereby improve outcomes by gathering, managing, and applying well-analyzed data. These skills are essential if DNPs are to rigorously evaluate innovative projects and if their work is to have impact.

In addition to introducing DNP students to the management of clinical and administrative data, including financial data, the book will be very useful for practicing DNP nurses and faculty.

The authors have intentionally designed a practical yet scholarly approach to analysis of clinical data and how to manage it. The book has been developed using their years of experience teaching in the DNP program at Johns Hopkins School of Nursing. The book reflects their cumulative learning through developing, implementing, and evaluating a novel approach to teaching clinical data management.

The chapters are arranged in a logical manner to build understanding and skills. Beginning with basic statistical concepts and power analysis, the reader is led through planning for data collection and developing an analysis plan, to data governance and creating the data set. The subsequent chapters address exploratory and outcomes data analysis; the concluding chapters focus on summarizing results of project evaluation and ongoing monitoring. Whether data are collected and analyzed for a specific project or gathered from multiple existing sources for a new project, these approaches are crucial if the project outcomes are to be credible.

The progressive case study illustrates multiple techniques and methods students can apply to their projects. More important, however, is the mastery of these techniques and methods for use by practitioners after graduation. The role of the practicing DNP requires an ability to translate evidence into practice in large organizations—that is, into clinical standards, quality improvement initiatives, and innovative management programs. DNPs with strong data management skills add value to organizations by documenting advances in clinical care, in the efficiency of care processes, and in the cost-effectiveness of programs.

Health care organizations are shifting from a fee-for-service model to a value-based model. Value-based health care focuses on costs, quality, and, most important, outcomes. The goal is high-quality and high-value care, with a reduced need for high-cost services. Central to this shift is the organization's ability to use data to measure the use of services, the quality of care, and patient satisfaction. The ability to define, measure, analyze, and demonstrate an improvement is central to the role of the DNP in health care's pursuit of value.

We are proud of the leadership and creativity Martha Sylvia and Mary Terhaar have demonstrated in designing courses, curriculum, and this book. They have carefully thought through the competencies needed by graduates of DNP programs if they are to fulfill their potential to be effective leaders of systems-level changes that will improve patient care and outcomes.

Martha N. Hill, PhD, RN, FAAN
Dean Emerita
Professor of Nursing, Medicine and Public Health
The Johns Hopkins University School of Nursing
Baltimore, Maryland

Karen B. Haller, PhD, RN, FAAN
Vice President for Nursing and Patient Care Services
The Johns Hopkins Hospital
Baltimore, Maryland

Preface

We are committed to the success of the DNP as a credential and to the success of the students who earn it. Our program prepares students to capably apply evidence to address important clinical problems and then evaluate the impact of their efforts. For 8 years we have taught students to adopt a posture of inquiry in their work, to use evidence to tackle important problems, and to rigorously evaluate their efforts. This approach prepares graduates to continually improve practice, to deliver outcomes, and to establish solid, credible programs of translation and improvement.

As faculty, we practice what we preach. We continuously evaluate the outcomes of our teaching and the work of our students. In that tradition, we conducted a review of the initial 38 capstone projects completed by DNPs in our program and determined that the evaluation component of the capstone needed to be more rigorous and data driven. In a review of the broader DNP curriculum, we identified and exploited opportunities to introduce content that would provide DNP students with the tools they needed to improve the data-driven components of the capstone project. Gap analysis revealed the need to strengthen plans for data collection, cleansing and manipulation, governance, analysis, and reporting. We decided to add an analytics course and set out to find a text to help us do so.

In the search for a text, we were surprised to find none that fully addressed the complexity of using clinical, operational, and financial data sets in various combinations to evaluate the impact of quality improvement and translation activities. Certainly, high-quality research and statistics texts are available and useful as a foundation for design and significance testing. Although essential, existing texts are not sufficient to prepare the DNP and other health professionals to translate evidence into practice and evaluate impact.

Absent a good text to guide the course, we set out to develop the content ourselves. Initially, Clinical Data Management (CDM) was offered as an elective, and course evaluations were favorable. More importantly, students who took CDM were more capable, comfortable, and independent in the analysis of their translation projects. We learned from their experiences, refined the course, and established CDM as a requirement for all DNP students. Evaluations improved, students succeeded and provided additional helpful feedback, and CDM was expanded to two courses in the second year of the program. Publications that resulted from the capstone projects increased, and graduates became increasingly successful in continuing the work of translation and evaluation they learned in the program. For example:

- Erik Southard used evidence and technology to provide consultation support to communities across rural Indiana, where psychiatric professionals are in short supply. He documented a decreased mean time to consult from 16.2 hours to 5.4 hours (Southard, Neufeld, & Laws, in press).

- Mariam Kashani and her colleagues added family risk and history of premature heart disease to risk assessment based on the Framingham Risk Score. As a result, 48% of 114 patients originally classified as low to moderate risk were reclassified as high risk, and 72% of those were found to have dyslipidemia, 35% had hypertension, 20% were prediabetic, and 61% evidenced atherosclerosis on carotid intima media thickness (Kashani, Eliasson, Vernalis, Bailey, & Terhaar, 2013).
- Lina Younan used evidence to establish handoff procedures that reduced errors of omission during intershift handoff ($n = 90$) from a mean of 4.96 errors per patient handoff at baseline to 2.29 per patient handoff postintervention ($p < .000$; Younan & Fralic, 2013).
- Bernadette Thomas made modifications to the electronic health record and used scorecards to increase chronic kidney disease screening (from 38% to 46%, $p = .049$), diagnosis (from 11% to 20%, $p = .000$), and use of appropriate medications among patients with diabetes (from 63% to 67%, $p = .000$) at a statewide federally qualified health center in Connecticut (Thomas, 2011).

All of these students tackled problems important to their organizations and communities. The analytics they applied allowed confidence in the conclusions they drew and all achieved statistically significant improvements.

This is the point at which we decided to write a text. We had developed content and a process useful to our students and faculty. We tested the text's value and reported an increase in capstone publications. We believe the content will be useful to others: to students, faculty leading other programs, and the organizations that employ DNPs. We want to share the evidence we collected to direct planning, gathering, entry, transforming, cleansing, governing, analyzing, and reporting of data. We invite schools of nursing with DNP programs that require scholarly projects to adopt and improve this process in support of establishing consistent, rigorous, well-evaluated translation. We want research to reach practical application expediently so the triple aims of quality, experience, and value can be attained (Berwick, Nolan, & Whittington, 2008) and so society can yield the return on its investment in basic research.

In the words of Charles-Guillaume Étienne, "One is never served so well as by oneself." We set out to write the text that could extend the success our students have earned. We hope it is helpful to all who seek to improve practice and outcomes through the judicious application of evidence and rigorous evaluation of the results.

Martha L. Sylvia
Mary F. Terhaar

REFERENCES

Berwick, D. M., Nolan, T. W., & Whittington, J. (2008). The triple aim: Care, health, and cost. *Health Affairs, 27*(3), 759–769.

Kashani, M., Eliasson, A., Vernalis, B. K., & Terhaar, M. (2013). Abstract 314: Systematic inquiry of family history improves cardiovascular disease risk assessment. *Circulation: Cardiovascular Quality and Outcomes, 6*, A314.

Southard, E., Neufeld, J. D., & Laws, D. (in press). Telemental health evaluations enhance access and efficiency in a critical access hospital emergency department. *Telemedicine and e-Health, 20*(7).

Thomas, B. (2011). Improving blood pressure control among adults with CKD and diabetes: Provider-focused quality improvement using electronic health records. *Advances in Chronic Kidney Disease, 18*(6), 406–411.

Younan, L. A., & Fralic, M. F. (2013). Using "best-fit" interventions to improve the nursing intershift handoff process at a medical center in Lebanon. *The Joint Commission Journal on Quality and Patient Safety, 39*(10), 460–475.

Acknowledgments

I would like to give a special thank you to everyone at Johns Hopkins Health-Care and Johns Hopkins University who have contributed to my clinical analytic journey: those who have mentored me, those who worked beside me, and especially those on my team of amazing analysts, past and present, from whom I learn every day. And to my husband Michael, thank you for all of your support and encouragement throughout this process.

Martha L. Sylvia

We want to recognize the community of scholars that is Johns Hopkins Nursing. It has been a once-in-a-lifetime opportunity to develop a new program in partnership with amazing educators, researchers, administrators, and clinicians. Each has made the program stronger and helped our faculty to develop students and curricula for the demands of care, quality, and value.

We thank Dean Hill for her courageous leadership. At a time when great uncertainty surrounded creation of a doctorate in nursing practice, Dean Hill challenged us to offer a program whose graduates would make Johns Hopkins University proud. She encouraged her faculty to lead, not follow, and her challenge freed us to undertake this work.

We especially thank our students for the challenges they present. The problems they undertake to solve press us to develop tools and processes to ensure both rigor and success. The populations they serve and the communities with whom they collaborate make great innovation possible. We celebrate your accomplishments and are pleased to contribute to your success.

Martha L. Sylvia
Mary F. Terhaar

CHAPTER 1

Introduction to Clinical Data Management

MARY F. TERHAAR

TRANSLATION

Timely application of strong science in the provision of direct patient care; management of health care systems; and education of clinicians, providers, and administrators are all compelling needs today in clinical data management (CDM). Science promises reduced suffering, improved quality of life, and increased productivity of individuals in societies. The challenge is to establish effective, disciplined mechanisms for translation that are accompanied by vigilant monitoring, rigorous analytics, and critical evaluation as innovation is brought to scale. These strategies are integral to delivering the innovation and reform that research findings proscribe, and every step on this path depends on data and analytics.

The purpose of this book is to describe a process and a set of strategies to be used to promote consistent, quality evaluation of the impact of translation. To adopt this approach builds a base of support for the work. This approach directs formation of a comprehensive plan that can be reviewed and approved prior to beginning any translation activity and then monitored throughout execution. It increases the quality of evaluation because it reduces error in data collection, measurement, and analysis. This, in turn, increases confidence of the team in its own potency, confidence of decision makers in the outcomes accomplished, and support within the organization for a program of translation. Because translation is central to the role of the Doctor of Nursing Practice (DNP), this text focuses on the DNP and presents examples of DNP work, data, and evaluations.

THE DOCTOR OF NURSING PRACTICE AS TRANSLATOR AND ANALYST

The DNP is a relatively new practice doctorate intended to improve outcomes for individuals receiving health care; for systems providing that care; and for professionals engaged in care, consultation, management, leadership, and the policy process. DNPs make their mark by accelerating the translation of robust evidence to improve outcomes. The value of the degree is judged by the results achieved.

The work of the DNP must be strong, scholarly, and significant. It must conform to accepted standards of researchers, clinicians, statisticians, and academics alike in order for the work to achieve its mark; the credential to endure; and for those who earn it to have lasting impact.

A set of core skills focusing on translation, collaboration, and evaluation is required for the DNP to be effective. Effective translation requires critical understanding and selection of evidence, careful planning, meticulous execution, reliable measurement, and robust evaluation. Knowledge of research design, program implementation, project management, statistics, epidemiology, professional and research ethics, data management, and analytics is the key (Sylvia & Terhaar, 2014).

THE CONTEXT OF DISCOVERY AND INNOVATION

Movement of science from the bench to the bedside brings significant change in context. Researchers formulate questions based on extensive study of existing knowledge; pose hypotheses for testing; control conditions in which these hypotheses are tested; select or develop measurement strategies that assure specificity and precision; and gather comprehensive data sets that ensure robust, generalizable conclusions can be derived. The hallmarks and the context of research are precision and control. Investigators maximize the effects of the variable(s) of interest, minimize the effects of extraneous variables, and control interactions known to impact the research question. The result is confident conclusions about relationships between variables and causality. The goal is new knowledge—discovery.

Translators operate in a different environment: the practice environment. They identify problems to solve, performance to improve, processes to refine, and conventions to question. Here, opportunity for innovation exists with minimal opportunity for control, and time is often critical. There is a calculus that seeks to minimize time to solution, as well as risk and error. Solution rather than discovery is the goal. Effective application of knowledge is the key.

Regardless of context and purpose, both research and translation require rigorous evaluation—the former to assure proper conclusions and generalizability of findings, the latter to determine applicability of research findings to a particular population and setting. This book provides a base of knowledge, describes the regulatory and ethical context, outlines a process to guide evaluation, presents a compendium of resources, and delineates examples of evaluation of translation efforts.

CLINICAL DATA MANAGEMENT

> [CDM is] [t]he process of planning, designing, collecting, cleansing, manipulating, analyzing, and reporting data generated in the assessment, development, delivery, and evaluation of health-related interventions, products, and services. (Sylvia & Terhaar, 2014)

Pharmaceutical companies employ CDM to evaluate sets of data from clinical trials (Lu & Su, 2010). Considered a distinct phase in clinical research by some, CDM produces reliable data and reduces time of a drug progressing from development, to trial, and ultimately to market (Krishnankutty, Bellary, Kumar, & Moodahadu, 2012).

Within the context of translation, CDM is most effectively seen not as a phase, but as a thread that crosses all activities of the work and promotes confidence in both process and outcome. Whether the work of teams, researchers, statisticians, or DNPs, CDM consistently refers to efficient and effective decision support using clean, reliable data.

The following paragraphs describe the procedures of CDM. Chapter by chapter, each introduces one component along with the foundational knowledge required for its deployment, tools to facilitate the work being described, and examples from translation projects.

Chapter 2: Basic Statistical Concepts and Power Analysis

In this chapter, the language of CDM is introduced and some elementary knowledge from statistics and research is reviewed. Types of measurement and levels of data are explained. Power analysis is outlined, emphasizing its critical importance to rigorous evaluation and manner of determination. Decisions about sample size and formation are presented in detail. Chapter 2 is not a statistics text, but a review of content vital to understanding the remainder of this book and to successful CDM in support of translation.

THOUGHTFUL PLANNING

Chapter 3: Preparing for Data Collection

Prior to completing the data analysis plan, a decision must be made about the sources of data to be used during the analytic phase of the DNP project. These sources are used to collect data for descriptive information and outcomes measurement. Feasibility, quality, specificity, and utility of primary data are compared to secondary data. Here, the logic for selecting either source is described and the implications for evaluation are reviewed.

Chapter 4: Developing the Analysis Plan

The first step in any data analysis is the creation of a data analysis plan that guides the entire project. A comprehensive process for planning analysis, including a description of considerations with respect to key decisions, is presented. Highlighted are the needs for descriptive data about the population, units of measurement, and the use and composition of comparison groups. In addition, outcome measures, calculations to derive scores, and other metrics are outlined. The construction and the sensitivity of measures that precisely evaluate the attainment of project aims are considered.

Chapter 5: Data Governance and Stewardship

The ethical responsibilities of those engaged in human subjects research are well understood and articulated. Although many in practice do not consider translation to be research, those who engage in this work need to adhere to the same requirements for protection of human subjects and peer review. Translators, like researchers, need do no harm. This chapter presents the critical importance of data governance and stewardship as one means to assure compliance with standards for professional ethics. The history, regulations, structures, and processes in place within each organization that impact the project, its execution, and the work of CDM are considered.

CAREFUL AND EFFECTIVE ACTION

Chapter 6: Creating the Analysis Data Set

High-quality results depend on high-quality data. This chapter explains the process of going from initial data collection or from the collection of secondary data to creation of a final analysis data set. This procedure includes importing data into statistical software, cleansing the data, manipulating the file and/or data, and creating a final analysis data set and data dictionary. Throughout the entire operation and any ongoing analysis, syntax is used as a method for documenting actions taken on the data and the decision process leading to those actions.

Chapter 7: Exploratory Data Analysis

Exploratory data analysis (EDA) is both a method for the investigation of data as well as a set of recommended tools and techniques with the fundamental tenet being that the data need to be explored and understood in their most basic form to the point of meaningful information (Smith & Prentice, 1993). This activity encompasses exploration of each variable individually and in meaningful combinations, as well as developing an understanding of the population and/or events of interest. It is necessary to carry out this EDA process prior to the analysis of outcomes measures. In conducting the EDA, the goal is to analyze data without expectations or assumptions. Thus, unexpected findings can be revealed. Chapter 7 considers the EDA as a strategy to create meaning from the collected data and to provide the structure and preparatory information needed to refine and execute the data analysis plan.

Chapter 8: Outcomes Data Analysis

Outcomes data analysis (ODA) is the final step in data management. Of all the phases of data management, ODA is perhaps the easiest after all the work that has gone into preparing and analyzing the data to this point. If the translational project does not use groups for comparison, then analysis of outcomes may be solely descriptive or may use a comparison to some type of benchmark or predetermined goal. If the translational project plan uses some type of comparison group, then statistical testing is done to determine the success of outcomes compared to another group or the same group at a different point in time. This chapter reviews execution of the analysis plan and evaluation of outcomes.

Chapter 9: Summarizing the Results of the Project Evaluation

Reporting of results is done within a defined structure; however, the content within that structure and the choice of format and mechanisms for delivery are chosen based on the primary interest of the target audience. Therefore, Chapter 9 describes the basic elements that need to be compiled for the reporting of results. Yet, variation is expected in the actual communication and presentation of this information based on the targeted audience and message.

Chapter 10: Ongoing Monitoring

Data management should be thought of as an ongoing feedback loop where data gathered, analyzed, and evaluated are used to continuously inform decisions and improve processes. As procedures are modified, deleted, or continued to achieve the desired outcome, the data must continue to be gathered and monitored to understand ongoing effects of the intervention and make decisions to further ensure that the best possible results are achieved. This chapter introduces the many tools that can be used to understand intervention techniques and outcomes, including statistical process control charts, run charts, and benchmarks. All of these can be used as part of broader, ongoing, continuous quality-improvement efforts to ensure that gaps in the intervention are met with effective responses and areas of weakness are addressed across the life span of the intervention.

CONCLUSION

The critical importance of improving practice and outcomes through the application of evidence has been significantly emphasized and resourced through collaborative efforts of the Robert Wood Johnson Foundation (RWJF) and the Institute of Medicine (IOM, 2010). Thousands of clinicians, educators, and administrators from around the globe have gathered to learn from experience, share strategy, and disseminate successes that target innovations and meaningful improvements in care, health, and cost (Berwick, Nolan, & Whittington, 2008). Scholarly journals, publications, and affiliations have developed the science and the practice of improvement and implementation. Johns Hopkins Hospital and its partners have cultivated processes and tools to be used by clinicians in the application of evidence in practice (Dearholt et al., 2012) and to support the work of translation (White & Dudley-Brown, 2012). Universities and clinicians providing direct care have designed models to promote timely, effective translation and system-wide collaborative change (Pronovost et al., 2006).

Health care professionals around the globe embrace the challenge of achieving the triple aim to improve performance: care experience, outcomes, and cost (Berwick et al., 2008). In presenting this treatise on CDM, the authors strive to set a standard for DNP practice that guides robust evaluation of the work of translation. If this new academic preparation of clinical nurse specialists, administrators, anesthetists, practitioners, midwives, informaticians, executives, and educators achieves its intended goal, the triple aim of improved care, health, and cost will be that much closer. Without meticulous CDM, this certainly remains out of reach.

REFERENCES

American Association of Colleges of Nursing. (2006). *DNP Roadmap Task Force Report.* pp. 1–80. Retrieved from http://www.aacn.nche.edu/dnp/roadmapreport.pdf

Berwick, D., Nolan, T., & Whittington, J. (2008). The triple aim: Care, health, and cost. *Health Affairs, 27*(3), 759–769.

Dearholt, S. L., & Dang, D. (2012). *Johns Hopkins nursing evidence based practice model and guidelines* (2nd ed.). Indianapolis, IN: Sigma Theta Tau International.

Institute of Medicine. (2010a). *The future of nursing: Focus on scope of practice.* Washington, DC: Author.

Institute of Medicine. (2010b). *The future of nursing: Leading change, advancing health.* Washington, DC: Author.

Krishnankutty, B., Bellary, S., Kumar, N., & Moodahadu, L. S. (2012). Data management in clinical research: An overview. *Indian Journal of Pharmacology, 44*(2), 168–172.

Lu, Z., & Su, J. (2010). Clinical data management: Current status, challenges, and future directions from industry perspectives. *Open Access Journal of Clinical Trials* (2), 93–105.

Pronovost, P., Needham, D., Berenholtz, S., Sinopoli, D., Chu, H., Cosgrove, S., . . . Kepros, J. (2006). An intervention to decrease catheter-related bloodstream infection in the ICU. *The New England Journal of Medicine, 355*(26), 2725–2732.

Smith, A. F., & Prentice, D. A. (1993). Exploratory data analysis. In G. Keren & C. Lewis, *A handbook for data analysis in behavioral science: Statistical issues* (pp. 349–390). Mahwah, NJ: Lawrence Erlbaum.

Sylvia, M., & Terhaar, M. (2014). An approach to clinical data management for the DNP curriculum. *Journal of Professional Nursing, 30*(1), 56–62.

White, K. M., & Dudley-Brown, S. (2012). Translation of evidence into nursing and health care practice. New York, NY: Springer Publishing Company.

CHAPTER 2

Basic Statistical Concepts and Power Analysis

MARTHA L. SYLVIA

Before embarking on the data management journey, it is important to review and have a good understanding of some basic statistics concepts and the methods of sample size determination. It is assumed that the Doctor of Nursing Practice (DNP) has taken a graduate-level statistics course, and it is recommended that a statistician be consulted for an examination of methods and development of more complex statistical models. This chapter discusses basic statistical concepts including types of variables, levels of measurement, and parametric and nonparametric statistical tests. Sample size determination methods that are applicable to the majority of DNP projects are described.

LEARNING OBJECTIVES

After reading this chapter, the DNP should be able to:

- Determine appropriate variable types and measurement levels for DNP data analyses
- Decide upon appropriate bivariate statistical test(s) to be used for measuring DNP project outcomes
- Apply the techniques of power analysis to determine an appropriate project sample size

REVIEW OF VARIABLE CONCEPTS

Types of Variables

Quality improvement and translation projects employ a variety of variable types for description and outcomes measurement. Variables differ according to the units of measurement and by the causal relationships between the variables being measured or investigated.

UNIT OF MEASUREMENT

Continuous variables are quantitative in nature. Theoretically they have an unlimited number of values and may or may not have a rational and meaningful value of zero. Those variables where a value of zero is possible are called ratio data. Weight is an example of a continuous measure at the ratio level. All arithmetic operations are permissible with ratio data because they have an absolute zero (Polit & Beck, 2012). Those variables where no absolute value of zero exists are at the interval level. Body temperature measured in the Fahrenheit scale is an example of interval data because it uses an arbitrary zero point (a value of zero does not indicate an absence of heat) (Polit & Beck, 2012).

Categorical variables, also known as discrete variables, have a limited number of values that can be named or classified. Some are nominal and others are ordinal. *Nominal* variables can be labeled or named but neither their sequence nor their relation to one another is meaningful. *Ordinal* variables, on the other hand, are so called because the sequence and the relationship of one value to another have meaning. Categorical variables can be counted and descriptive statistics can be used to describe their frequency of occurrence. *Dichotomous* variables are a type of categorical variable that is binary with two values (i.e., yes/no, gender). *Polytomous* categorical variables have three or more values (i.e., educational level, race; Plichta & Kelvin, 2013; Polit & Beck, 2012).

CAUSAL RELATIONSHIPS

The *independent* variable is the presumed cause or source of influence on the other variables of interest. In DNP projects it is usually a variable that indicates receipt of an intervention or the lack thereof. The *dependent* variable is the outcome or the presumed effect. It is the variable that will be impacted, or predicted. In DNP projects, the dependent variable is commonly abstracted from a data set created for the purpose of monitoring direct care (Polit & Beck, 2012).

Table 2.1 summarizes each type of variable, provides the definition along with examples, describes acceptable arithmetic operations, and lists the appropriate statistical tests for each level of measurement (nominal, ordinal, interval, and ratio).

BASIC STATISTICAL TESTS AND CHOOSING APPROPRIATELY

Understanding the type of variables to be managed makes it possible to select the appropriate statistical methods to be used for analysis. Nominal and ordinal variables do not lend themselves to the same analytics that can be used for interval and ratio data. Nominal and ordinal variables are best described by counting, and statistically tested using nonparametric methods. Interval and ratio variables are described using measures like means, ranges, and variations; they are statistically tested using parametric methods.

Nonparametric statistical tests do not depend on the assumption of normality of the data. Instead, these tests use ranking of the data and rely on the median as opposed to the mean. These methods are often used for testing nominal and ordinal data, when data do not meet the normality assumptions necessary for parametric testing, or with very small sample sizes (Plichta & Kelvin, 2013). Nonparametric tests are most commonly employed when data are skewed or when data are scores instead of measurements, such as Apgar scores, stages of disease, or visual analog scales (Altman, 1991).

TABLE 2.1   Definitions, Examples, and Descriptive Statistics for Different Variable Types

	Nominal	Ordinal	Interval	Ratio
Definition	Categorical variables measured only in terms of frequencies. Used to name, classify, or label.	Categorical variables that can be ranked or ordered according to degree. Known if a case has more or less of something but not the amount of more or less that it has.	Continuous, quantitative scale where the intervals between scores are consistent in magnitude. Arbitrary or nonexistent zero point.	Continuous, quantitative scale where the intervals between scores are consistent in magnitude. Difference is that there *IS* an absolute zero point.
Examples	Marital status, blood type, gender, race	Patient rating scales (pain, anxiety, depression, etc.), level of satisfaction, level of education	Blood pressure, temperature, body fluid measurement, lab values	Any measure in years, time, dollars, counts (pulse is ratio when measured as a function of time, i.e., beats/minute)
Descriptive statistics	Frequencies, percentages	Median, frequencies, percentages	Mean, median, mode, range, standard deviation, frequencies, percentages	Mean, median, mode, range, standard deviation, frequencies, percentages

Adapted from Polit and Beck (2012).

Table 2.2 provides information about nonparametric tests that may be useful for DNP project designs.

Parametric statistics are used with interval- and ratio-level variables. They are based on assumptions about the normal distribution of data and use means and standard deviations for calculations. When using a parametric statistical test, it is assumed and validated that the values for the dependent variable of interest are normally distributed. Occasionally a study will use parametric testing for ordinal data (this is often the case with Likert scales). Parametric tests are considered more powerful and flexible than nonparametric tests. Nonparametric tests are chosen as an alternative to parametric tests when the data under consideration cannot be construed as interval- or ratio-level measures or when the distribution of data is markedly abnormal (Polit & Beck, 2012). Table 2.3 shows information about parametric statistical tests commonly used in DNP projects, specifically the statistic used, and the purpose and the level of measurement for the independent and dependent variables. Chapter 8 provides more detail about interpreting the results of some of these tests.

SAMPLE SIZE CALCULATION USING POWER ANALYSIS

Power is the ability to determine statistical significance of the findings. Power analysis is the method used to determine the adequate number of subjects or events in each subgrouping of a population (note, population here refers to

TABLE 2.2 Nonparametric Statistical Tests

Statistical Test	Test Statistic	Purpose	Level of Measurement	
			Independent Variable	Dependent Variable
Mann-Whitney U test	U	Test the difference in ranks of scores of two independent groups	Nominal	Ordinal/interval/ratio
Median test	χ^2	Test the difference between the medians of two groups	Nominal	Ordinal
Kruskal-Wallis test	H	Test the difference in ranks of scores of three or more independent groups	Nominal	Ordinal/interval/ratio
Wilcoxon signed-rank test	Z	Test the difference in ranks of scores of two related or same groups	Nominal	Ordinal/interval/ratio
Friedman test	χ^2	Test the difference in ranks of scores of three or more related/same groups	Nominal	Ordinal/interval/ratio
Chi-square test	χ^2	Test the difference in proportions in two or more independent groups	Nominal	Nominal
McNemar's test	χ^2	Test the difference in proportions for paired samples	Nominal	Nominal
Fisher's exact test	–	Test the difference in proportions in a 2 x 2 table when $N < 30$	Nominal	Nominal
Spearman's rho	ρ	Test that a relationship exists	Ordinal	Ordinal
Kendall's tau	τ	Test that a relationship exists	Ordinal	Ordinal
Phi Coefficient	ϕ	Examine the magnitude of a relationship between two dichotomous variables	Nominal	Nominal

Adapted from Polit and Beck (2012); Polit and Hungler (1999).

the population defined within the data analysis plan) or number of events required to achieve statistically significant differences in results between groups, if they do exist.

DNP projects commonly seek to evaluate differences in outcomes between two groups, wherein members in one group receive care improved by translation of evidence (usually referred to as the intervention group) and members of a second group receive standard care (the comparison group). These groups, by necessity and design, are independent of each other. In some cases, however,

TABLE 2.3   Parametric Statistical Tests

Statistical Test	Test Statistic	Purpose	Level of Measurement	
			Independent Variable	Dependent Variable
t-test for independent groups	*t*	Test the difference between two independent group means	Nominal (two independent groups)	Interval/ ratio
Paired *t*-test	*t* (paired)	Test the difference between two related or same group means, usually at two points in time	Nominal (paired groups)	Interval/ ratio
ANOVA	F	Test the difference among the means of three or more independent groups	Nominal (three or more independent groups)	Interval/ ratio
Repeated-measures ANOVA	F	Test the difference among the means of three or more related groups, usually three or more points in time	Nominal (three or more linked groups)	Interval/ ratio
Pearson's product-moment correlation coefficient	r	Test the existence of a relationship between two variables	Interval/ratio	Interval/ ratio

ANOVA, analysis of variance.
Adapted from Polit and Beck (2012); Polit and Hungler (1999).

comparison of outcomes is conducted using the same group of subjects at two distinct points in time. This is usually referred to as pre/post-measurement in one group. It is important to note that for some DNP projects it may not be feasible to attain a number in each subgroup that is large enough to achieve statistical power; however, it is essential to know whether or not the subgroups were large enough and to be able to explain this when presenting the results of the project.

It is significant to clarify at this point that power analysis is a tool most often used in knowledge discovery research. Quality improvement and evidence translation projects often borrow from the tools of research in order to increase the rigor of evaluation. This use of power analysis to determine an adequate sample size is a meaningful tool in evaluating project outcomes and in providing more evidence that differences in outcomes between groups are actually due to the change in practice being tested (the intervention; American Psychological Association, 2009). Also, note that power analysis is used under the assumptions of parametric statistical testing; thus, except in the case of chi-square test of proportions, power analysis is not used when a nonparametric test is chosen.

The proper way to make a decision on sample size is to perform a power analysis, in the planning phase, prior to initiating any project. This is called "a priori" sample size determination and it is the ideal way to ensure that an adequate sample size is well thought out. Occasionally, a "post hoc" power analysis may be carried out after completing a project, when data are collected and analyzed and results have been determined. This is usually done to decide if the study was powered well enough to detect statistically significant differences between groups if they did exist in the absence of a priori determination. This type of analysis is considered controversial and is discouraged (Lenth, 2001).

Components of Power Analysis

Thinking about sample size calculation, it is important to understand the two types of errors that can occur when testing a hypothesized outcome. First, consider that when testing a hypothesized outcome, the real goal is to test if the assumption can be rejected that there is no difference between groups in the outcome measured. For example, in evaluating if there is a statistically significant difference in mean age between group 1 and group 2 (i.e., the mean age in group 1 is *NOT* equal to the mean age in group 2), the hypothesis would read:

$$\text{Mean age group 1} \neq \text{Mean age group 2}$$

However, the test of statistical significance is checking whether the opposite of the hypothesized outcome can be rejected. Investigation is done to see whether it can be rejected that mean age in group 1 is equal to mean age in group 2: the null hypothesis.

$$\text{Mean age group 1} = \text{Mean age group 2}$$

A power analysis and determination of adequate sample sizes are carried out to minimize the error that can occur in either rejecting the null hypothesis when it should not be rejected (Type I error) or accepting the null hypothesis when it should be rejected (Type II error). Table 2.4 helps to illustrate these errors.

Calculation of an adequate sample size is a factor of *significance level, statistical power, and effect size.* It is important to have sample sizes that are large enough to detect statistically significant differences in outcomes between groups when they do exist—but not so large that resources are used inefficiently in project implementation and data collection. In addition to the significance level, statistical power, and effect size, it is necessary to know the type of statistical test employed to determine the difference in outcomes (*t*-test [independent or paired], chi-square).

TABLE 2.4 Error Determination for Power Analysis

		In Actuality, the Null Is . . .	
		True	False
DNP/clinician decision about the null hypothesis	True (null accepted)	Correct conclusion 1-alpha (α)	Type II error 1-power beta (β)
	False (null rejected)	Type I error Significance level or alpha (α)	Correct conclusion Power or 1-beta (β)

SIGNIFICANCE LEVEL

In Table 2.4, the *significance level* or alpha is equal to the percentage chance that the null hypothesis is rejected when in actuality it is true. Said another way, this is the percentage chance of rejecting the null when the null is actually true, an incorrect conclusion or Type I error. This is the *p* level that is set in a study. It is usually set at $p = < .05$. This means that when $p = < .05$, there is less than a 5% chance that the null has been rejected (or that statistically significant differences among groups have been reported) when it should not have been.

STATISTICAL POWER

Beta equals the percentage chance that the null hypothesis is accepted when it is actually false. This is 1-power and is usually set at .20. This means that there is a less than or equal to 20% chance of accepting the null (or reporting no statistically significant differences between groups) when the null should have been rejected (and there really are statistically significant differences between groups). *Statistical power* is equal to 1-beta. It is the percentage chance of finding statistically significant differences between groups when they really exist. In other words, this is the percentage chance of rejecting the null when the null is actually false, a correct conclusion. Since beta is usually set at .20 or 20%, power or 1-beta is usually 80%.

EFFECT SIZE

The *effect size* is the magnitude or the *degree* to which the null hypothesis is false. This is the size of the effect desired in outcomes. An effect size can be determined in two different ways. The first is just a statement of the differences in means in the units of measurement desired (Lenth, 2001). For instance, a weight-loss intervention may seek to obtain a mean body mass index (BMI) that is at least 2 kg/m^2 less in the intervention group than in the comparison group (e.g., a mean BMI of 36 in the intervention group compared to a mean BMI of 38 in the comparison group). Another method standardizes the measure of effect across all outcomes, and Cohen's *d* is the most commonly used (Cohen, 1988). Cohen defines a small effect as 0.2, a medium effect as 0.5, and a large effect as 0.8. It is best to avoid estimating an effect size in sample size calculations by choosing a standardized effect size that is the "best estimate of the differences." The preferred method to decide effect size is to obtain the results of other similar studies measuring the same or similar outcomes (Lenth, 2001).

The formula for calculating the standardized Cohen's *d* effect size when testing the difference in means between two groups is:

1. The difference in two means: Effect size = d = $\dfrac{\text{(mean of group 1 } - \text{ mean of group 2)}}{\text{Estimated standard deviation of the overall population (sigma) or the standard error}}$

Note that when searching evidence to make estimations of the differences in means and standard error, often the standard error needs to be calculated using the standard deviation from previous studies. This is done by dividing the standard deviation by the square root of the sample size used in the study.

Figure 2.1 uses an example of differences in the Short Form 12 (SF-12) Physical Composite Score (PCS) values between an intervention and comparison group to show the interaction among all of these factors. In this example, the intervention group will be part of a program designed to increase mean PCSs. Based on existing evidence and current clinical information, it is expected that the comparison group will have a mean PCS of approximately 24 and the intervention group will have a mean value of approximately 42 (represented by the two mean lines at the center of each normal curve). The null hypothesis that will be tested is:

Mean PCS comparison group = Mean PCS intervention group

This is a two-tailed test (for the purposes of DNP projects, two-tailed test assumptions are appropriate) and is depicted by α/2 in each of the light gray of the comparison group normal curve. Alpha (α) is the percentage chance of committing a Type I error or saying that there is a statistically significant difference in PCS levels between the intervention and comparison groups when there really isn't a difference. This risk of a Type I error is divided in half between the two tails of the curve. Power (1-β) is represented by the area filled with dashed lines. Beta (β) is the area in dark gray, and it is the percentage chance of committing a Type II error or determining that there is no statistically significant difference in PCSs when there really is a difference. (Note that the placement of power, beta, and α/2 is depicted as it is currently, with an expected increase in the score. If the expected change were a decrease, the graphs would be flipped or opposite their position in Figure 2.1.)

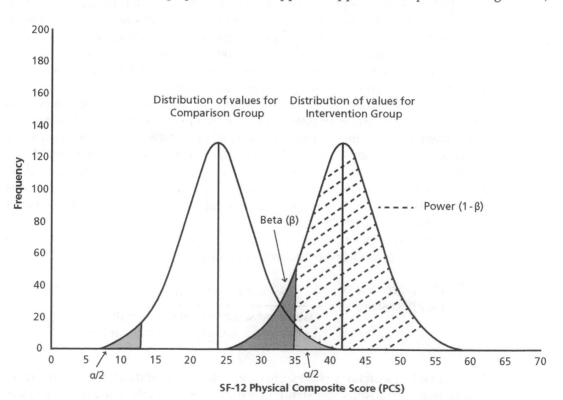

FIGURE 2.1   **Example of interaction of factors used to determine sample size in power analysis.**

Sample Size Determination for Paired Data

This section describes the considerations for sample size when observations are paired and outcomes are measured using continuous data (the paired t-test is the statistical test of choice here). Testing differences in means for paired data, the concepts are similar to those in testing independent group means—with the disparity being that each individual prevalue is subtracted from the postvalue and the mean of those differences is then compared to zero. The standard deviation used in determining effect size is the standard deviation of the mean of the differences (Altman, 1991). This method is similar to the independent t-test in the way that mean contrasts are compared; however, variance is usually lower in the paired t-test because of the correlation in pre/post-measurement inherent in the design of using the same individuals (Paired Difference Test, 2013).

For example, in testing, if the mean of all the values of (weight 2 – weight 1) are statistically significantly different from zero, the hypothesis would read:

$$\text{Mean of (weight at point 2} - \text{weight at point 1)} \neq 0$$

However, the test of statistical significance is checking whether the opposite of the hypothesized outcome can be rejected. Analysis is conducted as to whether the mean of all the values of (weight 2 – weight 1) is equal to zero can be rejected: the null hypothesis:

$$\text{Mean of (weight at point 2} - \text{weight at point 1)} = 0$$

Sample Size Determination for Proportions

This book describes sample size determination for proportions under certain assumptions that are more common in problems addressed by the DNP. The first assumption is that the two groups being tested are independent (i.e., the proportions are not being measured in the same group of individuals at two separate points in time), or stated another way: The observations are independent (one outcome or observation per individual). (Note, if a study of proportions is needed for paired data, the nonparametric McNemar's test should be used.) Next, it is assumed that the dichotomous outcome of interest is not a rare event (e.g., death). The last assumption is that the two groups being evaluated have equal numbers of individuals (in the planning phase, it is understood that by the end of project implementation there may be slight differences in the numbers in each sample).

Hypothesis testing for proportions follows the process similar to testing in means. Expanding on the previous hypothesis testing example for means, if instead of looking at differences in mean age the inquiry was to determine whether there was a significant difference in the percentage of individuals over the age of 65 in one group compared to another, the hypothesis would be stated as:

$$\text{Proportion of individuals in group 1} \geq 65 \neq \text{Proportion of} \\ \text{individuals in group 2} \geq 65$$

The test of statistical significance is investigating if the opposite of the hypothesized outcome can be rejected. The statistical test is conducted to see whether it can be rejected that the proportion of individuals in group 1 ≥ 65 is equal to the proportion of individuals in group 2 ≥ 65: the null hypothesis.

Proportion of individuals in group 1 ≥ 65 = Proportion of
individuals in group 2 ≥ 65

With adequate sample sizes, a sample proportion has an approximately normal distribution. Thus, if the sample size and proportions are not very small, the concepts for calculating sample sizes in proportions are similar to those for continuous data or testing the differences in means (Altman, 1991).

Influence of Other Factors on Sample Size

- Sample size *increases* as significance (alpha) *decreases.*
- Sample size *increases* as power (1-beta) *increases.*
- Sample size *decreases* as the effect size *increases.*

Using Sample Size Calculators

Once the conceptual basis of sample size determination is understood, one of the many helpful online sample size calculators can be utilized. Here are some of the websites that can be used:

- www.stat.uiowa.edu/~rlenth/Power
- www.stat.ubc.ca/~rollin/stats/ssize
- statpages.org
- www.biomath.info/power/index.htm
- statpages.org/proppowr.html
- www.biomath.info/power/chsq.htm
- www.biomath.info/power/prt.htm

Many statistics and research textbooks also have sample size calculation tables as appendices. This is another way to decide upon sample size. Additionally, some statistical software like Stata and SPSS have sample size calculators. For the purposes of this book, Russ Lenth's work is used (first item on the list of websites above; Lenth, 2006–2009). This calculator can be downloaded as software or utilized online. Because of its interactive nature, the calculator is ideal for determining the effects of small changes in each of the inputs. (Note: It is important to consult with a statistician for guidance, review, and approval of the sample size calculation. However, it is equally essential for the DNP to understand the sample size calculation!)

TWO INDEPENDENT GROUPS: COMPARING MEANS

Employing sample size calculators to determine the difference in means between two independent groups, the elements needed are: (a) the type of statistical test performed to compare the differences in the two means—in this case, the two-sample *t*-test or the independent *t*-test; (b) the expected difference in means;

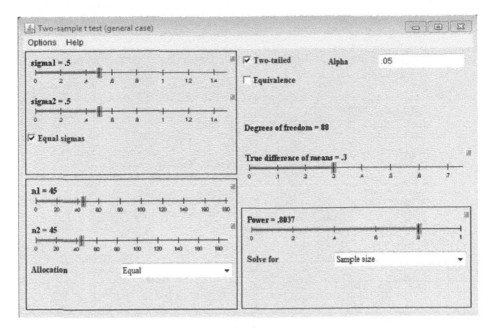

FIGURE 2.2   Sample size calculation for independent means.

Output obtained using Lenth (2006–2009).

(c) the expected standard deviation of the mean in each group (input as sigma 1 and 2 in this calculator); (d) the significance level or alpha; and (e) power.

In the next example (Figure 2.2), an independent *t*-test is used to determine if there are statistically significant differences between an intervention group that received a program to improve HbA1C levels and a comparison group that did not receive the program.

In this illustration, the following information is determined and known:

- Alpha = .05
- Power = 0.80
- Previous evidence shows, with this intervention, HbA1C difference between intervention and comparison patients is:
  - Mean comparison = 7.5
  - Mean intervention = 7.2
  - Standard deviation in each group = 0.5
    - (Note, this calculator requests the expected standard deviation in each group to determine variance so that the standard error does not need to be calculated manually.)

PAIRED GROUPS: COMPARING MEANS IN ONE GROUP AT TWO MEASUREMENT POINTS

Applying sample size calculators to determine the difference in means in the same group at two separate measurement points, the elements needed are: (a) the type of statistical test performed to compare the differences—in this case, the one-sample *t*-test or the paired *t*-test; (b) the mean of the differences between pre/post-individual values—in this calculator stated as True [mu-mu$_0$]; (c) the expected

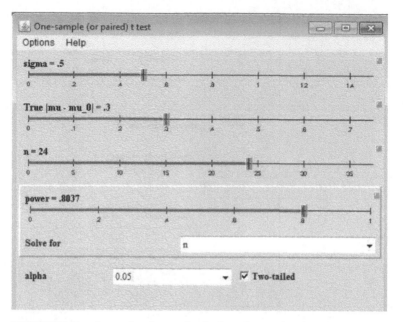

FIGURE 2.3   Sample size calculation for paired means.
Output obtained using Lenth (2006–2009).

standard deviation of the mean of the differences between individual pre/post-values (input as sigma in this calculator); (d) the significance level or alpha; and (e) power.

In the example in Figure 2.3, the following elements are known:

- Alpha = .05
- Power = 0.80
- Previous evidence shows, with this intervention, HbA1C differences pre/post-measurement are:
  - Mean of differences in pre/post-values = 0.3
  - Standard deviation of mean of difference in pre/post-values = 0.5

Notice that when entering the same values for power, significance level, difference in expected means, and difference in standard deviation, the sample size required for a paired design is lower than for the design using independent comparison groups. This is because of the inherent correlation between the two measurements for each individual in the paired design. Also note that the power is not exactly 80%: The calculator moves the decimal point in power slightly to provide a whole number for the sample size.

TWO INDEPENDENT GROUPS: COMPARING PROPORTIONS

Using sample size calculators to compare proportions, it is only necessary to enter the expected proportion in each group. The standard error is a calculation based on these two proportions; therefore, the sample size calculator can make that determination as part of the calculation. Sample size calculators usually provide an option for a sample size determination with and without continuity correction.

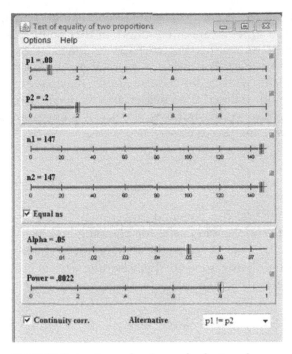

FIGURE 2.4   Sample size calculation for proportions.
Output obtained using Lenth (2006–2009).

The methods use a normal distribution to approximate the binomial distribution for dichotomous data. It is wise to use the sample size determination with the continuity correction for a more conservative estimation of sample size and especially when the samples are small (Altman, 1991).

In the example in Figure 2.4, the following elements are known:

- Alpha = .05
- Power = 0.80
- Previous evidence shows, with this intervention, the difference in the proportion between intervention and comparison patients who show an improvement in their HbA1C is:
  - $p_1 = .08$
  - $p_2 = .20$

Often, a DNP project has more than one outcome—some that may compare means and others that may compare proportions. Additionally, there may be a paired design component and an independent design component within the same project. The priority is usually to ensure that there is power on the most important result(s). If all outcomes are equally vital, it is wise to determine sample size using the conclusion that requires the largest sample sizes. This usually falls into the following order of tests: (a) proportions, (b) independent means, and (c) paired data means.

Regardless of the type of measurement for outcomes, the best way to determine the expected differences in means, standard deviations, and/or proportions is to reference previous peer-reviewed research evidence that has reported the results of a similar intervention in a similar population. Often, however, evidence that meets these criteria cannot be found; at that point, peer-reviewed research evidence that is similar to—but perhaps somewhat different from—the current project may be used. For instance, an intervention used to improve self-management in patients with cardiovascular disease may have similar results when used in patients with asthma. If no evidence is available, decisions about expectations should be grounded in clinical experience. It is important to estimate the input factors for power analysis as closely as possible.

SUMMARY

An understanding of statistical concepts and power-analysis methods for determining sample size is a crucial prerequisite for planning and executing a data-analysis plan. Armed with this knowledge, the DNP is able to choose appropriate variables and statistics and decide upon adequate sample sizes in order to answer complex clinical questions using data.

REFERENCES

Altman, D. G. (1991). *Practical statistics for medical research.* Washington, DC: Chapman & Hall/CRC.

American Psychological Association. (2009). Criteria for the evaluation of quality improvement programs and the use of quality improvement data. *American Psychologist, 64*(6), 551–557.

Cohen, J. (1988). *Statistical power analysis for the behavioral sciences.* New York, NY: Lawrence Erlbaum.

Lenth, R. V. (2001). *Some practical guidelines for effective sample-size determination.* Iowa City, IA: University of Iowa Press.

Lenth, R. V. (2006–2009). Russ Lenth power and sample size calculator [Computer software]. Java Applets for Power and Sample Size. Retrieved June 12, 2013, from http://www.stat.uiowa.edu/~rlenth/Power

Paired Difference Test. (2013, May 19). Retrieved June 22, 2013, from https://en.wikipedia.org/wiki/Paired_difference_test

Plichta, S. B., & Kelvin, E. (2013). *Munro's statistical methods for healthcare research* (6th ed.). Philadelphia, PA: Lippincott Williams & Wilkins.

Polit, D. F., & Beck, C. T. (2012). *Generating and assessing evidence for nursing practice* (9th ed.). Philadelphia, PA: Lippincott Williams & Wilkins.

Polit, D. F., & Hungler, B. P. (1999). *Nursing research: Principles and methods.* Philadelphia, PA: Lippincott Williams & Wilkins.

CHAPTER 3

Preparing for Data Collection

MARTHA L. SYLVIA

P rior to completing the data analysis plan, a decision must be made about the sources of data to be used during the analytic phase of the Doctor of Nursing Practice (DNP) project. These data sources are used to collect variables utilized for descriptive information and outcomes measurement. Important factors that are vital to this decision include the feasibility of collecting primary data compared to repurposing existing secondary data; the quality and usefulness of the selected data source; and the precision with which the variables within the chosen data source can match the desired measure. Once a data source is chosen, the data structure and mechanisms for collecting the data must be determined.

LEARNING OBJECTIVES

After reading this chapter, the DNP should be able to:

- Explain the benefits and limitations of using primary and secondary data sources
- Determine primary and secondary data sources
- Decide upon the appropriate data source for the DNP project

PRIMARY AND SECONDARY DATA

Definition

DNPs collecting data for a project have a choice of whether to use primary or secondary data sources. Primary data are data collected at the time of and specifically for the purpose of measuring some type of descriptive or outcome information for the DNP project/intervention. Some examples of primary data include pre/postpatient or staff knowledge tests; focus-group responses; intervention checklists; or surveys to measure satisfaction, confidence, perceptions, or other specific project outcomes. Secondary data sources are those that have been collected for a purpose other than the DNP project/intervention, and may or may not have been collected at the same time as the project implementation. Examples of secondary data sources include data collected from patient-monitoring devices, administrative claims data submitted for billing, laboratory results, health care provider assessments, electronic medical record (EMR) data, and care plan data. Primary and secondary data have both advantages and disadvantages that need to be considered when making the decision about which to use; often the DNP chooses to use data from both types of sources to measure project results.

Deciding Which Data Sources to Use

Many factors go into determining whether to use primary or secondary data. The first major decision point is whether or not data sources exist to measure what is necessary to meet the requirements set forth in project aims and outcomes. If data are already available and being collected, the quality of that data must be assessed to conclude whether it meets the informational needs of the project. One important aspect of assessing quality is determining the completeness of the available data. To calculate completeness, an appraisal can be done on a small subset of the data to determine the amount of missing data. For instance, in a specific DNP project, one of the measures was to judge if a certain cholesterol laboratory value was within a desired range for a group of patients with cardiovascular disease. In order to determine if the laboratory result data, which were available through a vendor contract with the health plan, could be used for measuring this program outcome, an analysis was undertaken to assess completeness. The laboratory vendor data containing laboratory results was compared to the laboratory billing data for services to determine the percentage of bills for laboratories that could *not* be matched to a service in the laboratory vendor result data. During this analysis it was concluded that 40% of the bills for a laboratory service could not be matched to any laboratory results. This amount of missing data was not tolerable for measuring the outcomes for the DNP project and another solution using primary data sources had to be arranged.

Another aspect of secondary data source quality is data cleanliness. This relates to the research terms of reliability and validity. For the purposes of assessing secondary data, reliability is the competence of the data collection mechanism to *consistently measure what it is intended to measure*. The key to reliability is consistency or the ability to produce the same results under consistent conditions. Measurement of weight is a good example because weight measurement is stable within moments in time. A reliable calculation of weight would produce the same result for weight, regardless of the number of times measured over a short time frame. It is best to explore a sample of the secondary data and look at the distributions of the data when determining the reliability of a secondary data source. Look for erroneous values (e.g., a blood glucose reading of .20 or 3450). Also, check for differences in measurement units: If weight is usually measured in pounds and there is a weight value of 75 lbs. for an adult man who is 6 ft. tall, it may be that some of the entries are in pounds and some are in kilograms. See the section on data cleansing in Chapter 6 for more details.

Another way to assess the reliability of the data is to observe the data collection process. This method is useful when employing data that can be assumed by the collector or stated by the patient (e.g., race can be assumed by the nurse from making a judgment based on skin color or other patient features, or the nurse can ask the patient directly); are collected in a format that requires manual entry (e.g., the nurse entering blood pressure and weight information); or are subjectively collected (e.g., data from fields in provider or nurse assessments and care plans for patients). In one DNP project example, a process measure of "assessing for tobacco use" was going to be calculated from the secondary data source of the nurse case manager intake assessment within the patient-centered medical home. This intake assessment was completed for every patient but by a team of five staff nurses. The DNP observing the staff nurses performing the intake assessment found that the question to patients was not worded consistently. In some cases, nurses asked patients if they used tobacco and in other cases they asked patients if they smoked. Additionally, the same nurses would not always ask the patients at all—assuming the answer to the question based on their knowledge of the patients and therefore filling in the information without inquiry.

Validity is the degree to which what is intended to be measured is actually being measured. A very clear-cut example is a fetal heart-rate monitoring device that is valid when it is actually calculating the fetal heart rate and not the mother's heart rate. Validity becomes more complex in measuring emotions, feelings, and perceptions—as in the cases of satisfaction scores, pain severity, self-management of illness, stages of change, etc. It is important to keep in mind, when assessing secondary data for validity, the data collection mechanism was created for a purpose other than the particular project at hand. Using secondary data sources, validity is a very significant consideration because the data source chosen must address the specific aim and outcome of the project. Often, usually due to feasibility, a data point is chosen to calculate a specific outcome that does not *exactly* measure what the aim of the project is intended to impact.

The best way to assess the validity of secondary data sources is to determine if the validity and reliability of the data collection tool used have been published either in the scientific peer-reviewed literature or by the manufacturer of the device or instrument. Another evaluation of validity needs to be undertaken by the DNP leading the project to decide if the data collection device/tool/instrument was intended to measure and is measuring what is within the DNP's project aims and results. The following DNP project provides a good example of the nuances of this type of validity assessment. This project was put in place to improve care coordination for all the patients with severe chronic illness in the Accountable Care Organization (ACO) by assigning each patient a nurse case manager. One of the aims was to improve patient satisfaction. As part of the operations of the ACO, a satisfaction survey was mailed to patients every 6 months. Due to feasibility issues in administering a separate satisfaction survey, the DNP wanted to use the data from the ACO satisfaction survey to determine an improvement in patient satisfaction. However, on closer examination of the ACO satisfaction survey, 75% of the questions were focused on satisfaction with the primary-care provider. Therefore, it was not likely that the survey would measure an increase in satisfaction due to the care coordination intervention.

Following this assessment of data quality, the trade-offs must be considered. The quality appraisal gives a good idea of the state of the secondary data that are already available for meeting the measurement needs of the DNP project. The results of the quality evaluation need to be weighed against the feasibility of collecting primary data. The two main reasons for collecting primary data as opposed to using secondary data are: (a) the data point that must be measured does not exist in any secondary data sources, and (b) the quality of secondary data is too poor to meet the needs of measurement for the DNP project evaluation. Collecting primary data, however, is usually a much more resource-intensive undertaking in terms of establishing data collection mechanisms, determining data collection tools, and data entry. Data collection mechanisms refer to the structure in which the data are collected. To illustrate: A database may have to be developed; an existing data system (e.g., an EMR) may need to be modified; or an online survey tool may have to be configured. Data collection tools may require permissions to use any proprietary validated instruments or, if nonexistent, will require development. If extensive, data entry may necessitate additional staff or much of the time of the DNP leading the project.

Table 3.1 summarizes the trade-offs to be considered when making the decision of whether to use primary or secondary data sources.

TABLE 3.1   Considerations for Primary and Secondary Data Sources

	Primary Data Sources	Secondary Data Sources
Applicability to purpose, aims, and outcomes of project	Directly applicable	May not be directly applicable; proxy may need to be considered
Timing of data collection	At the time of the project implementation	May or may not be at the time of the project implementation
Data collection mechanism	Requires creation of new mechanisms or modification of existing data collection systems	Already established
Data collection instruments	Requires determination and/or development of collection tool	Already established
Data entry	Requires resources to perform data entry	Already completed
Completeness of data	Usually fully complete due to control over collection	Needs to be assessed; likely less than 100% complete
Reliability	Usually high due to control over implementation of data-collection processes	Needs to be assessed; likely compromised
Validity	Usually high due to control over choice of measurement instrument	Needs to be assessed; trade-offs may be necessary

USING PRIMARY DATA

Reliability and Validity of Data Collection Instruments

It is best to use data collection instruments, whenever possible, that have established reliability and validity. Reliability and validity were discussed earlier in this chapter in assessing the data quality of secondary data sources; however, in this section reliability and validity are defined in the context of selecting data collection instruments for primary data collection. In terms of data collection devices such as blood pressure cuffs, scales, blood glucose monitors, etc., the manufacturer of the data collection instrument should provide information about validity and reliability. Additionally, the Food and Drug Administration's (FDA) Center for Devices and Radiological Health is responsible for regulating firms that manufacture, relabel, and/or import medical devices sold in the United States. The FDA maintains a database of all approved devices and their associated validation studies (U.S. Department of Health and Human Services, 2013).

Survey instruments selected for primary data collection should have established reliability and validity published in either peer-reviewed scientific literature or in organizational white papers. As opposed to the peer-reviewed scientific literature, white papers contain written information about a survey tool and are created by a business to help the consumer understand the detailed specifications of the tool. White papers are more rigorous when validation studies within the white paper and the white paper itself are written by experts external to the organization. It is preferable and more scientifically exacting to choose data collection survey tools that have published reliability and validity in the peer-reviewed literature. Least desirable is the creation of a survey instrument by the DNP for the purposes of the project at hand. Although it may be necessary to create questions that capture factual or obvious descriptive information such as age, numbers of years of X, gender, presence of disease conditions, etc., if the concepts being measured are more complex—satisfaction, pain, confidence, readiness to change, etc.—then validity and reliability should be established for the chosen instrument.

Reliability is the extent to which an instrument yields the same results in repeated administrations (Writing @ Colorado State University, 2013). Interrater reliability, a determination of whether two or more observers are consistent in their perceptions, should be assessed any time a person observer is responsible for measurement. Interrater reliability is evaluated by determining the percentage agreement between two observers. Test–retest reliability is assessed by appraising the Pearson correlation coefficient between two administrations of the same test to the same individuals at two different points in time. Judgment of internal consistency reliability uses Cronbach's alpha to calculate the degree of correlation among questions that were designed to measure the same construct within an instrument (Web Center for Social Research Methods, 2006). In these measures of reliability, usually a value of 0.8 or greater is desirable.

Validity is the extent to which the instrument measures what it is intended to measure, as opposed to reliability—representing the accuracy of the measure. Face validity is a common-sense look at the results by experts in the field to determine whether it makes sense that the instrument measures what it is supposed to measure. Criterion validity compares the results of one instrument to another validated measure of the same or similar concept. For instance, a new subjective tool to assess for depression might be tested in those with and without an established diagnosis of depression. Construct validity assesses the agreement between a theoretical concept and the measurement of that concept, and requires a great deal of thought in defining a concept. Content validity evaluates the extent to which an instrument measures the intended domain of content (Writing @ Colorado State University, 2013). The design of instrument-research studies to appraise validity varies depending on the constructs and measurement of those constructs and the type of validity being determined. Therefore, it is important to carefully read and interpret validation studies when choosing a measurement instrument.

Data Collection Mechanisms

ONLINE SURVEY TOOLS

Survey tools that are available online offer a fast and flexible way to gather, measure, and sometimes even analyze survey data. Online survey tools should meet these basic functionality requirements: secure and easily accessible data storage; online interface for building survey questions; the ability to send a link for the survey to potential survey respondents; and ease in exporting survey data for analysis. Many survey tools are available for free; however, some companies providing tools charge a fee that is usually associated with more sophisticated functionality of the survey and/or support from an expert in survey development. Consider, when choosing a free account, that many online survey tools place limits on the number of questions, surveys, and responses possible under this arrangement. Additional valuable functions to think about include:

- The ability to personally brand the survey without the survey company name being prominently displayed.
- The skill to offer the survey in multiple languages.
- Limited or no advertising for the respondent when opening, taking, or exiting the survey.
- The competence to use *skip* logic so that respondents do not have to answer unnecessary questions. Skip logic allows the survey developer to determine whether a subsequent question should be answered based on the response to a current question.
- The ability to require answers from respondents for certain questions.
- Being able to assign an ID number to a respondent that can be used later to link survey data to other data sources (e.g., clinical data, administrative claims data) or to a future administration of a survey (e.g., pre/post-test of knowledge).
- The skill to use *piping*, which allows the survey developer to incorporate the response from a previous question into a current question. For instance, if participants answered that they did not get an appropriate health screening this year, the current question could query the type of assistance that might be necessary for them to get the health screening.
- The ability to randomize the question order. This is helpful when administering a knowledge test, to discourage respondents from answering together with other participants.

- The competence to embed a survey within a webpage separate from the survey tool company webpage. This is useful if the organization has its own website where potential respondents are already accessing information and services.
- The ability to analyze data in the survey tool itself. Whereas this can be very useful, if this function requires a charge for use of the tool, it may be more beneficial to move the data into a statistical software package for analysis (Leland, 2011).

Table 3.2 gives a listing of common online survey tools that are helpful for DNP projects, and provides information about important considerations when making a choice among these tools.

TABLE 3.2 Available Online Survey Tools and Considerations for Their Use

Survey Tool	Web Address	Free Basic Version?	Complex Functions Offered?	Considerations
Survey Face	www.surveyface.com	Yes	Yes/free	A large amount of functionality for free with unlimited questions, responses, and surveys
Survey Moz	www.surveymoz.com	Yes	Yes/cost	Good functionality for free with limits on questions and responses
SoGo Survey	www.sogosurvey.com	Yes	Yes/cost	Limits on free functionality; advanced functions with range of costs
Survey Monkey	www.surveymonkey.com	Yes	Yes/cost	Basic functionality limited; higher cost for more advanced features
Zoomerang	www.zoomerang.com	Yes	Yes/cost	Basic functionality limited; higher cost for more advanced features
Survey Gizmo	www.surveygizmo.com	No	Yes/cost	Advanced features with range of costs
Poll Daddy	www.polldaddy.com	Yes	Yes/cost	Limits on free functionality; advanced functions with range of costs
PsychData	www.psychdata.com	No	Yes/cost	Advanced features with expert support at various cost options

(continued)

TABLE 3.2   Available Online Survey Tools and Considerations for Their Use (*continued*)

Survey Tool	Web Address	Free Basic Version?	Complex Functions Offered?	Considerations
Qualtrics	www.qualtrics.com	No	Yes/cost	Sophisticated features to support multiple research designs in industry and academics
Question Pro	www.questionpro.com	Yes	Yes/cost	Advanced features with expert support with range of costs
Lime Survey	www.limesurvey.com	Yes	Yes/free	Free and powerful open-source software; requires IT development support
Key Survey	www.keysurvey.com	No	Yes/cost	Most robust; highest cost

Adapted from Leland (2011).

Regardless of the brand of survey tool used and the level of available functionality, a great deal of thought and planning need to go into the design of the survey. It will be up to the DNP or designee to design and develop the survey. If the survey tool used is one that has been validated in the literature, the survey items need to be written into the online survey tool as is—ideally with no changes to the original. Additional questions may need to be added into the online survey for informational needs beyond the study itself (e.g., age, gender, and other demographic data). Much more preparation in design is necessary for a survey that is being developed specifically for the project at hand. In this case, it is better to write the survey questions on paper or in an electronic document prior to programming them in the online survey tool.

MANUAL DATA ENTRY

Online survey tools allow exporting of data to statistical or spreadsheet software for analysis; however, when survey administration is on paper or when data points are being collected at the point of care, appropriate software is required for data entry and preparation for later examination.

Although there are many software options available, Microsoft Access, Microsoft Excel, and IBM SPSS are the three most common options used by the DNP. A database organizes information around the person or event for which data are being collected. Microsoft Access software allows the creation of a data-collection database with a moderate learning curve. It permits multiple data tables with a linking ID among tables. This is beneficial when the project requires multiple data sets, with some having many records per person/event and others having one record per person/event. For example, one table might house demographic information such as age, gender, disease state, etc. for a patient; another table might hold a record for each hospital admission for each patient listed in the demographic table. The database allows all this information to be contained within the same structure and to be linked by the patient ID. Once data are entered into the database, retrieval can be accomplished by querying or asking pertinent questions; filtering and sorting the information; and producing reports from the database tables combined in ways determined by the user.

Databases provide a big advantage over spreadsheet documents. They allow multiple users to enter data at the same time, and the data entered are saved in real-time if everyone is accessing the same database from the same server location (this may require remote access to the server where the database is located, if those entering the data are not all in the same physical location). This advantage means that there is no need for version control—as is the case when using spreadsheets—and therefore much less risk of losing data. Despite the benefits of databases for data entry, DNPs may reject this option because the learning curve is higher than that necessary for spreadsheets and it may require some technical assistance. If possible, however, a database is a more secure and less risky choice for data collection.

Spreadsheet software such as Excel allows the entry of data in rows and columns in one spreadsheet per data source. For example, entering the responses from survey data of patients, each row would be a patient and the columns would represent survey responses. One disadvantage of spreadsheets is that they do not easily allow for multiple responses to a single survey question. A column must be set up for each possibility of the multiple responses with a *yes* or *no* value for each possibility. Another disadvantage is that more than one person cannot use the same Excel spreadsheet at the same time. It quickly becomes very cumbersome to manage many versions of spreadsheets and adds a higher risk of losing data. Spreadsheet software supports calculations and statistical analysis during the data collection process. This is useful in checking the quality of data entry while the project is ongoing.

Data from both Access and Excel are directly importable into SPSS software for statistical analysis. Sometimes the DNP may choose to enter data directly into an SPSS data sheet. SPSS is more sophisticated than Excel in its ability to link and merge information from multiple data sets but it is not database software. Therefore, it has some of the same risks inherent in using Excel because there is a higher risk of losing information when multiple users are entering data. Statistical software does, however, permit data cleaning, manipulation, and some analysis during project implementation. This is useful for checking data quality and performing some preliminary exploratory data analysis prior to project completion.

MODIFICATION OF EXISTING DATA COLLECTION SYSTEMS

Many health care organizations have well-established information systems that are used for business operations. Most of these systems are configurable in that assessments, surveys, care plans, and/or additional questions, etc. can be added with minimal effort. The added benefit is that these systems are already being used by the clinical staff involved in the DNP project implementation. As opposed to asking staff to complete separate data entry requirements, placing the required data entry fields into the existing clinical system where staff members already work makes it easy to incorporate these fields as part of existing work flows. Modification of an established system usually requires support and prioritization from the organizational IT department.

USING SECONDARY DATA

Sources of Secondary Data

REGIONAL HEALTH INFORMATION ORGANIZATION (RHIO)

An RHIO is a type of health information exchange organization that brings together health care stakeholders within a defined geographic area and governs health information exchange among them for the purpose of improving health and care in that specific region. RHIOs typically include participating health care provider organizations, payers of health care services, laboratories, public health departments, and hospitals. A board of directors made up of stakeholders from each of the types of organizations provides governance over the RHIO and makes decisions about which data to share and the mechanisms for sharing that data (U.S. Department of Health and Human Services, 2005). In some states, the RHIO is actually a statewide health information exchange (HIE).

Despite U.S. government investments in HIE, there is limited exchange of health information with health care providers in outpatient settings; long-term care facilities; rehabilitation faclities; and other health care organizations outside of hospitals. The most prevalent source of data being exchanged comes from acute-care settings with information about hospitalizations (U.S. Department of Health and Human Services and Centers for Medicare and Medicaid Services, 2013). In order to understand if data that may be suitable for a DNP project are available within a RHIO, it is important to define the boundaries of the RHIO within which the patient population data would be housed, and determine the types of data available within that RHIO. This information can be found by performing an Internet search for HIEs in the location of interest.

ELECTRONIC HEALTH RECORD (EHR)

The EHR is a longitudinal electronic record of patient health data generated by one or more encounters in any care-delivery setting. EHRs include information about patient demographics, progress notes, medical problems, medication prescriptions, vital signs, past medical history, provider/nurse assessment of health status, care plans, immunizations, laboratory data, and radiology reports (Health Information and Management Systems, 2013).

The patients for whom EHR data are available are those receiving their services within the health care organization for which the EHR is in place. An EHR can serve a population as small as those seen by one health care provider or as large as those seen by an entire ACO or academic health institution. It is crucial to know if patients' documentation for the entirety of their health care services is within the same EHR. It is common, for instance, for a patient to receive primary-care services under one EHR and receive specialist services within a different health care organization with a different EHR or charting structure. Additionally, patients may travel for a portion of the year and receive health care services in various parts of the country.

HEALTH RISK ASSESSMENT (HRA)

An HRA is an evidence-based tool that is used to assess the health status of individuals through self-reported responses to health-related questions. Although HRAs may vary, common areas of assessment within an HRA include chronic condition and cancer disease risk, family history, nutritional status, fitness level, stress level, mental health status, substance use, safety risks, follow-up of medical conditions, use of preventive health examinations, self-perception of health status, readiness to change risky health behaviors, and absenteeism or lost productivity at work or at school (Vigil & Sylvia, in press).

HRAs are most often administered by employers and health insurance plans to manage the health risks of the populations for which they hold some type of risk for payment of health care services. The information is commonly used to offer employees or health insurance beneficiaries access to programs and services to improve their health and remove health risks. When using HRA data, it is important to understand the population in which it is offered; the percentage of potential respondents who actually complete the HRA; and any other possible limitations on the offering of the HRA that may present a bias in the data. For example, some self-insured employers only offer the HRA to employees and not to the dependents of employees who may be receiving health benefits under the same self-insured health insurance plan.

ADMINISTRATIVE MEDICAL CLAIMS DATA (MCD)

Administrative MCD contain the information that is submitted on a bill to a payer of health care benefits for medical services. For the most part, the payer is usually either the U.S. government by way of the Centers for Medicare and Medicaid Services or a health insurance company. However, the receiver of MCD can also be a third-party administrator (TPA). A TPA administers claims payment mainly for self-insured employers. In these cases, payments for health care services are made on a fee-for-service basis—payment is determined and distributed to providers based on the service received by the patient. When health care services are paid on a fee-for-service basis, there is a standard form used across all billing provider organizations. The information available in MCD that is useful for project evaluation includes patient demographics, medical diagnoses, date of service, place of service, type of service, procedure performed, provider of service, type of provider performing the service, billed amount by the provider, paid amount by the payer, and any copayment by the patient. Each type of clinical information uses standardized coding systems. For instance, medical diagnosis coding uses the *International Classification of Diseases, Ninth Revision, Clinical Modification (ICD-9-CM)* coding system.

In some cases, payment is not based on the service received but is instead based on a rate that is *capitated*—one payment is made to the provider of services that covers a range of possible services supplied to the patient. Another scenario where payment may not be made for services received is in the case of a health maintenance organization like Kaiser Permanente or such as within the Department of Veterans Affairs (VA). In these cases, there may or may not be administrative MCD available.

Administrative MCD have an advantage—the payer for the patient is usually the same regardless of which provider the patient sees for which type of service. Therefore, the MCD from the payer of services for a patient will contain all the medical claims data available for that patient. So, for instance, when determining costs per patient, MCD contain all the costs per patient and provide a complete measure of costs. Utilizing MCD, it is important to understand the benefit package and copayment information for the patient population. There are many varieties of options of benefit structures and copayments that affect the completeness of information available for a patient. It is also significant to comprehend the length of time each individual in the patient population has been enrolled in the health plan. If unfamiliar with MCD, it may be helpful to get assistance in using these data for project evaluation.

ADMINISTRATIVE PHARMACY CLAIMS DATA (PCD)

Administrative PCD are similar to MCD with regard to the payer/provider structure, except that the provider is a pharmacy. It is also the norm for pharmacy claims to be paid by the prescription filled. Information within PCD that is useful for project evaluation includes patient demographics; fill date; prescribing physician; pharmacy filling the prescription; National Drug Code (NDC)—a 10-digit number that incorporates information about the drug manufacturer, drug strength, drug form (or route of delivery), and packaging; days of supply of the medication; and cost to the payer and patient.

The payer of PCD for a patient may or may not be the same payer as the MCD for the same patient as is the case when a patient has one health insurance company for medical care and a different prescription drug insurer. If they are paid by the same payer, the combination of PCD and MCD provides a rich source of information about patients in a population. PCD should be given the same patient-based considerations as MCD, and an expert in using these data should be consulted regarding variable creation and methodology. Most payers have analytic departments in place that regularly work with these data for quality and accreditation reporting purposes.

BILLING DATA (BD)

BDs have many of the same elements as MCD and PCD. The big difference is that the underlying population for which the data exist is the one receiving services from the provider organization or pharmacy that is doing the billing. This is opposed to MCD and PCD, where the underlying population is all the individuals insured by the health plan or other payer. BD can be useful when the data and measures for the underlying population for project evaluation need only come from one organization. An example would be when a hospital wants to measure the change in costs or length of stay for a particular procedure during implementation of a quality-improvement initiative.

LABORATORY VENDOR DATA (LVD)

LVD hold information about the laboratory service supplied to patients when they have a provider-ordered lab test performed. LVD are different from the data contained in administrative claims data about a lab because they contain detailed information about the lab test itself and its results. Laboratory information in medical claims data only have that which is necessary for payment of the service. LVD typically include but are not limited to data about patient demographics, date of lab test, type of lab test, health plan enrollment or payer, ordering physician, diagnosis for lab test (important to note that this is not necessarily a confirmed patient diagnosis but may be a rule-out diagnosis), type of test, industry standard logical observation identifiers names and codes (LOINC) to identify results of test, accepted range for the result, and an indicator of an abnormal result.

LVD can be obtained directly from the laboratory vendor, but more often providers and payers of health care services have contracted with lab vendors to provide regular files of lab results. Therefore, lab result data are usually available for both provider and health plan affiliated patients and can likely be combined with other sources of data.

DEVICE MONITORING DATA (DMD)

Over the past 5 to 10 years, a plethora of DMD have become available from multiple sources, including hospital monitoring systems like cardiac and vital sign devices; remote chronic condition monitoring through the use of telemonitoring call-in, web-based, and actual personal devices like weight scales and blood pressure cuffs; and smartphone health monitoring applications. Although there is not a great deal of experience in using some of these data sources, they are important to consider as part of an evaluation of DNP projects. To illustrate, one DNP project used a smartphone application to collect patient-reported stress outcomes while implementing a stress-reduction program. The application monitored physical symptoms as well as patient perception (*BP Magazine*, 2012). The sources of DMD vary and, especially if collected by a private company, there are often challenges with access to the data because of ambiguity about the ownership and use.

Table 3.3 highlights some of the data elements that are important for measurement in DNP projects and shows which data sources of those described are *ideal* for obtaining each element.

Requesting Secondary Data From an Organization

First, before inquiring for secondary data from an organization, it is vital to understand the organizational policies and processes for releasing data and the procedure for requesting data. Some organizations have formal policies in place, whereas others do not. It is beneficial to have an advocate who can help with navigating the process within the organization. Second, it is essential to have an organized and thoughtful request written out that can be shared as a working document with staff at the organization who complete the data request. The staff members who complete a data request are usually technically skilled, and not clinically trained, data programmers. Therefore, they generally complete the inquiry *exactly* as requested. It is crucial to communicate the requirements of the request in as much detail as possible; which will prevent multiple iterations of the request and inefficient use of technical resources for querying. The data management plan described in Chapter 4 serves as a good structure for data request, and can be used as is to accompany any formal query an organization may already have in place.

SUMMARY

Data collection requires a thoughtful plan prior to execution of the DNP project. The use of primary versus secondary data sources and the benefits and costs/risks must be weighed into the decision of which source to employ. It is also critical to consider data quality, reliability, and validity. A well-developed plan for acquiring data allows for ease of data collection and analysis during and after project implementation.

TABLE 3.3 Ideal Data Sources for Important DNP Project Data Points

Potential DNP Data Points of Interest for Project Evaluation	Ability to *Ideally* Retrieve From Each Data Source							
	RHIO	EHR	HRA	MCD	PCD	BD	LVD	DMD
Patient demographic information								
Age, gender, race, etc.	Yes	Yes	Yes	Yes	Yes	Yes	Yes	Varies
Past medical history	No	Yes	Yes	Varies	No	Varies	No	No
Family medical history	No	Yes	Yes	No	No	No	No	No
Event descriptive information	Yes	Yes	No	Yes	Yes	Yes	Yes	Varies
Patient-reported health perception/ behaviors								
Perceived health status	No	Yes	Yes	No	No	No	No	Varies
Readiness to change	No	Yes	Yes	No	No	No	No	Varies
Activation	No	Yes	Yes	No	No	No	No	Varies
Knowledge	No	Yes	Yes	No	No	No	No	Varies
Symptoms	No	Yes	Yes	No	No	No	No	Varies
Functional status	No	Yes	Yes	No	No	No	No	Varies
Exercise habits	No	Yes	Yes	No	No	No	No	Varies
Nutritional intake	No	Yes	Yes	No	No	No	No	Varies
Alcohol, drug/tobacco use	No	Yes	Yes	No	No	No	No	Varies
Worksite health and safety	No	Yes	Yes	No	No	No	No	Varies
Stress and coping status	No	Yes	Yes	No	No	No	No	Varies
Access to medical care	No	Yes	Yes	No	No	No	No	Varies

TABLE 3.3 Ideal Data Sources for Important DNP Project Data Points (*continued*)

Potential DNP Data Points of Interest for Project Evaluation	Ability to *Ideally* Retrieve From Each Data Source								
	RHIO	EHR	HRA	MCD	PCD	BD	LVD	DMD
Patient health outcomes								
Prevalence of illness/comorbidity	Varies	Yes	Yes	Yes	Yes	Yes	Yes	Varies
Laboratory results (e.g., HbA1C, LDL, etc.)	Varies	Varies	No	No	No	No	Yes	Varies
BMI	No	Yes	Yes	No	No	No	No	Varies
BP	No	Yes	Yes	No	No	No	No	Varies
Medication adherence	Varies	No	No	No	Yes	No	No	Varies
Nurse-sensitive outcomes (Ingersoll, McIntosh, & Williams, 2000)								
Satisfaction with care delivery	No	No	Varies	No	No	No	No	Varies
Symptom resolution/reduction	No	Yes	No	No	No	No	No	Varies
Perception of being well cared for	No	No	Varies	No	No	No	No	Varies
Compliance/adherence	No	Yes	Varies	Yes	Yes	Yes	No	Varies
Knowledge of patients/families	No	No	No	No	No	No	No	No
Trust of care provider	No	No	No	No	No	No	No	Varies
Collaboration among care providers	No	Yes	No	No	No	No	No	No
Care-provider recommendation according to need	No	Yes	No	Varies	Varies	Varies	No	No
Frequency and type of procedures	Yes	Yes	No	Yes	No	Yes	No	Varies
Quality of life	No	Yes	Yes	No	No	No	No	Varies

(continued)

TABLE 3.3 Ideal Data Sources for Important DNP Project Data Points (*continued*)

Potential DNP Data Points of Interest for Project Evaluation	Ability to *Ideally* Retrieve From Each Data Source							
	RHIO	EHR	HRA	MCD	PCD	BD	LVD	DMD
Utilization and cost types								
Hospital admissions; length of stay	Yes	No	No	Yes	No	Yes	No	No
Hospital readmissions	Yes	No	No	Yes	No	Yes	No	No
ER visits	Yes	No	No	Yes	No	Yes	No	No
Primary care/specialty care visits	Varies	Yes	No	Yes	No	Yes	No	No
Use of laboratory/radiology	Varies	No	No	Yes	No	Yes	Yes/Lab	No
Durable medical equipment	No	No	No	Yes	No	No	No	No
Medications prescribed	Varies	Yes	No	No	No	No	No	Varies
Medications filled by patient	Varies	No	No	No	Yes	Varies	No	Varies
Dialysis visits	No	No	No	Yes	No	Yes		
Long-term/postacute care services	Varies	No	No	Yes	No	Yes	No	No
Hospice services	Varies	No	No	Yes	No	Yes	No	No
Vision and dental services	No	No	No	No	No	No	No	No

BD, billing data; BMI, body mass index; BP, blood pressure; DMD, device monitoring data; EHR, electronic health record; ER, emergency room; HbA1C, hemoglobin A1C; HRA, health risk assessment; LDL, bad cholesterol level; LVD, laboratory vendor data; MCD, medical claims data; PCD, pharmacy claims data; RHIO, regional health information exchange organization.

REFERENCES

bp Magazine. (2012, July 26). Need to reduce stress? There's an app for that. Retrieved July 22, 2013, from https://bphope.com/Item.aspx/994/need-to-reduce-stress-theres-an-app-for-that

Health Information and Management Systems. (2013). *HIMSS. Electronic health records*. Retrieved July 15, 2013, from http://www.himss.org/library/ehr/?navItemNumber= 13261

Ingersoll, G. L., McIntosh, E., & Williams, M. (2000). Nurse-sensitive outcomes of advanced practice. *Journal of Advanced Nursing, 32*(5), 1272–1281.

Leland, E. (2011, February). *Idealware. A few good online survey tools*. Retrieved July 14, 2013, from http://www.idealware.org/articles/fgt_online_surveys.php

U.S. Department of Health and Human Services. HRSA Health Information Technology and Quality Improvement. (2005). *What is a regional health information exchange?* Retrieved July 14, 2013, from http://www.hrsa.gov/healthit/toolbox/RuralHealthITtoolbox/ Collaboration/whatisrhio.html

U.S. Department of Health and Human Services. U.S. Food and Drug Administration. (2013, June 20). *Medical devices*. Retrieved July 13, 2013, from http://www.fda.gov/ MedicalDevices/default.htm

U.S. Department of Health and Human Services and Centers for Medicare and Medicaid Services. (2013, March 3). Advancing interoperability and health information exchange. *Federal Register: Daily Journal of the United States Government*. Retrieved July 15, 2013, from https://www.federalregister.gov/articles/2013/03/07/2013-05266/ advancing-interoperability-and-health-information-exchange

Vigil, I. M., & Sylvia, M. L. (in press). Health risk assessment. In S. Kahan, A. C. Gielen, P. J. Fagan, & L. W. Green (Eds.), *Health behavior change in populations*. Baltimore, MD: Johns Hopkins University Press.

Web Center for Social Research Methods. (2006, October 20). *Types of reliability*. Retrieved July 12, 2013, from http://www.socialresearchmethods.net/kb/reltypes.php

Writing @ Colorado State University. (2013). *Reliability and validity*. Retrieved July 12, 2013, from http://writing.colostate.edu/guides/page.cfm?pageid=1386

CHAPTER 4

Developing the Analysis Plan

MARTHA L. SYLVIA

MARY F. TERHAAR

The first step in any data analysis is the creation of a data analysis plan. This plan serves as a guide throughout an entire project. It (a) defines the data elements to be collected; (b) provides a structure within which to collect that data; and (c) outlines the analytic steps needed to identify, interpret, present, and disseminate final results to analytic questions that are important to Doctors of Nursing Practice (DNPs).

LEARNING OBJECTIVES

After reading this chapter, the DNP should be able to:

- Describe the unit(s) of measurement for data analysis
- Determine comparison groups
- Define descriptive and outcome variables
- Develop outcomes, measures, and calculations for each project aim

APPLYING THE ANALYSIS QUESTION

Fully developed analysis questions of the DNP usually fall into two categories: descriptive or evaluative. Descriptive questions are generally asked when trying to understand a problem or other phenomena, a population or event, an organization, etc. For instance, a DNP might seek to understand the characteristics of a population in order to determine the fit of a solution found in the evidence to a particular population, or the descriptive analysis might help to evaluate the feasibility of a potential intervention. When the purpose of a data analysis is evaluation, the question(s) are expressed as aims and outcomes. For example, the evaluation of an intervention designed to improve health outcomes for obese people might seek to answer the outcome question: "Did people exposed to the intervention achieve the weight-loss goals?"

DETERMINING THE UNIT OF ANALYSIS

The analysis plan begins with a detailed description of the unit of analysis that usually falls into one of two categories: population or events. A population is made up of people, and may include patients, staff, nurses, physicians, etc. (Note that the definition of "population" in this text is limited to that available for the DNP evaluation of a specific project and is not meant to equate to the statistical definition of "population" to which generalizations are made.) A population is chosen as the unit of analysis typically when trying to understand something about the experience of individuals; in this case, each individual should be counted only once in the overall measurement. The second category—events—is the occurrence of some type of activity or delivery of a health care service or procedure. Some good illustrations of events include laboratory draws, visits to a clinic, hospitalizations, readmissions, change-of-shift handoffs, etc. The units of analysis provide structure for the evaluation and both label and define the rows of data in the evaluation data set.

The decision of whether the unit of analysis is a population or an event depends on the analysis question of interest. For instance, a question might focus on establishing the number of individual patients who were assessed for having received an influenza shot during hospital admission. In this case, each patient would be counted only once to determine if there had been an assessment. The unit of analysis in this case could be expressed as "patients admitted to the hospital unit during the month of June," and if a patient had more than one admission during June, that person would only be counted once. However, in ascertaining the rate of assessment for influenza per admission, the unit of analysis would be each unique hospital admission during June—regardless of whether a patient had been admitted twice or more during that month.

Sometimes the unit of analysis is events that occur at several points in time, which can lead to the creation of a longitudinal data set. This is often the case when using monitoring data to measure some type of outcome and can include data points such as vital-sign readings, alarm alerts, administrative claims data points (i.e., cost and utilization), patient contacts/phone calls, etc. Longitudinal data sets are important to create when the desire is to understand the details of each event as it occurs without the information being summarized or aggregated in any way. These types of detailed observations can be very cumbersome to manage; however, they are worth the effort because they can provide a much richer understanding and more granular answers to the analysis questions.

For instance, in comprehending the costs of providing care for a population over a period of a year, the unit of analysis can begin at varying levels of hierarchy. The unit of analysis could be each individual claim submitted for payment for a defined group of patients during the year. In this example the unit of analysis is individual claim lines. At this level of analysis a great amount of detail can be gleaned about the costs associated with each data point—the procedure administered, the place and date of service, and the provider administering the service. Alternatively, the unit of analysis could be an aggregated monthly cost figure for a group of patients during the year; in this case the unit of analysis would be a monthly observation of costs for each patient (12 rows per patient). At an even more highly summarized level, the unit of analysis could be the total sum of the year's cost for each individual in the analysis. Here, the unit of analysis would be the patient, and one of the variables in the data set would be the costs for the year. The last two choices do not allow as detailed an understanding about the nature of the costs as does the first selection.

Creating Comparison Groups

Comparison groups are useful to construct when the analysis question is evaluative in nature. The purpose of using a comparison group is to decide whether outcomes have been successfully met by comparing two groups of similar individuals (or events). There are multiple approaches to creating comparison groups that may be considered for DNP projects, including random group assignment, pre/post-comparison of the same individuals over time, causal comparison group, similar comparison group in the postperiod, or comparable comparison group in both the pre/post-period.

The most rigorous way to compare groups is to use random group assignment. Randomization means that placement of individuals within a group is done using a method that ensures every person has an equal chance of being assigned to each grouping (Polit & Beck, 2012). Random assignment is the best way of ensuring that groups are equal to each other in demographic and other characteristics (although there is no guarantee) so that the effect of an intervention can be attributed to the intervention itself instead of one of these characteristics. Randomization is not usually feasible for the translational interventions of the DNP for varying reasons, including (a) feasibility, it may not be financially or structurally possible to assign groups indiscriminately; (b) ethical considerations, translational interventions are often provided to all who qualify; and (c) program evolution, translational projects may follow rapid-cycle improvement methods or organizations may undergo structural and/or procedural changes (Ovretveit & Gustafson, 2002).

A comparison group that is created in a causal comparison design is one that occurred under similar circumstances and has attributes similar to the intervention group; however, all measures and outcomes occurred at a previous point in time when the intervention did not exist. For example, a DNP project might seek to increase the response time to abnormal laboratory values and use, as a comparison, a set of abnormal lab values that occurred a year prior to the intervention to measure follow-up time.

The comparison group can also be the same group of people but at different subsequent points in time—pre/post-comparison. This method is commonly used when testing improvement in knowledge in patient and/or staff and provider education interventions. The pre/post-comparison group is not used when the unit of analysis is an event because the same event cannot be measured at two points in time.

Another way to create a comparison group is within a context where a similar group of individuals (or events) have not been exposed to the intervention. This matching group is created so that measurement can take place in both a preperiod and postperiod that would allow looking at the "differences in differences"—which compares the difference between the preperiod and postperiod outcome in each group and determines whether this difference is more favorable in the intervention group. Alternatively, a comparison group can be created so that the differences in postintervention measures can be compared at the end of the intervention. In either case, it is important to create a situation where the comparison group is as similar as possible on as many attributes as likely, as well as to ensure that the groups have similar exposure to all contextual factors except for the intervention. For example, in a DNP project where the goal was to reduce readmissions for a group of older patients at risk for a fall, the intervention group was exposed to a nurse transition guide intervention. A comparison group was created of seniors at risk for a fall who were cared for in a similar setting but without the nurse transition guide. The differences in fall rates pre/postintervention were compared for the two groups.

When using methods other than random selection of assigning a comparison group, there is a greater risk of introducing bias or confounding into the measurement of successful outcomes. This is because the comparison group may be heterogeneous or different from the intervention group on some dimension or characteristic. To illustrate, if the comparison and intervention groups significantly differ in mean age, then the results of an outcome could be due to this difference in age instead of receipt of the intervention. The use of pre/post-measurement in the same group over time can remove the bias that could be found due to differences between the memberships of each group. However, there can be bias in postmeasurement—due to familiarity with the content area and questions—if the group is given the same test. This bias is less of a problem in same-group pre/post-measurement when using objective outcomes measures as opposed to self-reported measures. Using a differences in differences approach, as is the case in the similar comparison group in the pre/post-period, provides much stronger evidence that outcomes are attributable to the project intervention when randomization cannot be used (Ovretveit & Gustafson, 2002). Although there is not as much control over bias or confounding in creating nonrandomized comparison groups, techniques can be used to adjust for differences between groups when measuring outcomes. These strategies are covered in Chapter 8.

Elements Used to Describe the Unit of Analysis

Certain elements are necessary when describing the unit of analysis. These include:

- Subgroupings (comparison groups) of the overall population/collection of events
  - These are important when the analysis question is evaluative, outcomes are compared between two or more groups, or results are evaluated within one group at different points in time.
- Source(s) of data for identification
  - The source is the origin, location, and/or purpose for generating the data.
  - This is the source of data that is used to create inclusion and exclusion criteria for the population or events.
- Number expected
  - The number expected quantifies the total membership or inclusion in the group, population, or aggregate of events to be understood or evaluated.
  - This number includes the breakdown by any subgroupings. To ensure that statistical significance, if it exists, is found in outcomes, this number is based on a sample size determination using power analysis (see Chapter 2). Sometimes it is not feasible to include a number high enough to achieve statistical power but it is important to know whether or not an evaluative analysis question is powered.
- Inclusion criteria
  - The inclusion criteria define the rules by which an individual or event is included in the population and any subgroupings.

TABLE 4.1 Example of a Population as Unit of Analysis

Name of the population	Employees with chronic conditions
Subgroup receiving program intervention	Full-time employees of units A, B, and C
Subgroup for comparison	Full-time employees of units D, E, and F
Source(s) of data	Employee health plan enrollment and administrative claims data
Number expected	Approximately 240 members in each subgroup
Criteria for inclusion	▪ Employed full time for at least 1 year ▪ 18 years of age or older ▪ Presence of at least one chronic condition from health care claims data ▫ Diabetes, cardiovascular disease (CVD), asthma, chronic obstructive pulmonary disease(COPD)
Criteria for exclusion	▪ Anyone currently receiving treatment for cancer (identified in health care claims data)
Time frame	The population is identified if it ever met the criteria during the past 3 consecutive years starting in January of the current year

- Exclusion criteria
  - The exclusion criteria detail the rules by which an individual or event meeting all of the inclusion criteria would *not* be included. Exclusion criteria are *not* the opposite of inclusion criteria.
- Time frame for identification
  - This is represented by dates and defines the time period in which the population is identified. Other information that is collected about the population or events may or may not be gathered during the same time period that data about the population/event are assessed to determine inclusion and exclusion. For example, when identifying a population of patients with asthma, the population may have had a diagnosis of asthma in the previous year; however, demographic and outcome information about that population would likely be collected in an upcoming year.

Table 4.1 shows an example of a population description, and Table 4.2 shows an example of event description using each of these elements.

DETERMINING THE VARIABLES OF THE DATA SET

After defining the unit of analysis or "rows" of the data set, the analytic plan then moves to defining the "columns" or variables in the data set. The variables that make up the columns of the final data set fall into two categories: descriptive or demographic, and outcomes. Descriptive information is any documentation that helps explain significant characteristics of the population or collection of events. If the analysis question of interest is solely descriptive, then the data plan is complete with using descriptive information. However, if the question of interest is evaluative, the variables necessary to measure outcomes need to be determined. Outcomes data include any variables that assist in measuring the final project results.

TABLE 4.2   Example of an Event as Unit of Analysis

Name of the event	Intershift handoffs at a hospital
Events exposed to the program intervention	Handoffs in units A, B, and C
Events used for comparison	Handoffs in units D, E, and F
Source(s) of data	Handoff documentation log, recordings of handoff
Number expected	Approximately 300 member handoffs in each group
Criteria for inclusion	▪ Handoff must occur between two registered nurses ▪ Handoff occurs at change of shift
Criteria for exclusion	▪ Unrecorded handoffs
Any special populations to consider in measurement?	▪ Identifier for each handoff and receiving RN ▪ Identifier for patient discussed at handoff
Time frame	Handoffs are measured during the 4-month period of current year, from April 1 to July 31

Descriptive Information

Descriptive information can include variables that may be related to or impact outcomes in an evaluation. For instance, there may be significant age differences between two subgroupings of a population that affect the conclusion of an outcome. It is important in this phase of planning to give careful thought to information that needs to be collected, to decide if there are any biases in subgroupings that may affect outcomes at the end of an evaluation.

The first step in gathering descriptive information is to assign a unique identification number to each member of the population or each event. This is vital because it is a reminder of the uniqueness of each row in the data set and it allows for linkages among multiple data sets containing data on the same individuals or events. Unique identifiers also allow for necessary data manipulation and analytical functions in the data analysis phase.

Descriptive information for a population of people falls into two main categories specific to either the person or the context.

- Person-specific information includes variables such as:
  - Age
  - Gender
  - Race
  - Diagnosis
  - Income category
  - Education level
- Context-specific information includes variables such as:
  - Hospital unit
  - City, state, zip code
  - Number of procedures
  - Time of day
  - Exposure to radiation

TABLE 4.3 Example of Descriptive Variable Information

	Variable Name	Variable Description	Data Source	Possible Range of Values	Level of Measurement	Time Frame for Collection
POPULATION	EmployeeID	Unique assigned identification number		N/A	Text	Onset of intervention
	Age	Age at start of intervention	Health plan enrollment data	18–100	Continuous	Onset of intervention
	Gender	Gender		1 = female 0 = male	Dichotomous	Onset of intervention
	Yrsemployed	Today's date minus employment start date		1–60	Continuous	Onset of intervention
	Radexpose	Indicator of whether employee had exposure to radiation	Employment health record	1 = yes 0 = no	Dichotomous	Any exposure during employment
EVENT	HandoffID	Unique assigned handoff number		N/A	Text	At time of handoff
	Shift	Shift in which handoff occurred		1 = day 0 = night	Dichotomous	At time of handoff
	Unittype	Description of hospital unit	Handoff log created for this project	0 = medical 1 = surgical 2 = pediatric 3 = oncology	Nominal	At time of handoff
	NurseID1	Badge number of nurse handing off patient		N/A	Text	At time of handoff
	NurseID2	Badge number of nurse receiving patient		N/A	Text	At time of handoff

N/A, not applicable.

Descriptive information for a collection of events also falls into two main categories related to either the event or the context.

- Event-specific information includes variables such as:
  - Date
  - Time
  - Unit/department
  - Method of procedure
  - Brand of equipment
- Context-specific information includes variables such as:
  - Patient identifier
  - Nurse identifier
  - Physician identifier
  - Family members present

Information about the descriptive variables should include:

- Variable name
- Variable description
- Data source
- Range of values possible
- Level of measurement
- Time frame for collection

Table 4.3 illustrates an example of descriptive variable information for the population and set of events described in Tables 4.1 and 4.2.

Outcomes Information

Given that a translation project is conducted to improve outcomes, an outcome statement is derived from the project aims and defines success. An example of an outcome statement might be: "There are 25% more patients in the intervention group, as compared to the comparison group, who have received their flu vaccine." In this instance, the independent variable is the grouping variable (intervention or comparison) and it is an indicator of receipt of an intervention to improve flu vaccine administration. The dependent variable in this illustration is the receipt of the flu vaccine, and it is dichotomous. This book assumes that outcomes measures are chosen that are appropriate for the project purpose and aims. Thus, it does not go into sources of or choosing appropriate outcomes measures.

Measures are derived from the outcome statement and explained in terms of the specific dependent variable and the calculation to be performed on that variable (i.e., usually a mean or percentage). A measurement statement describes how the outcome is quantified within this particular project and contains the variable to be measured as well as the way it is to be measured. An example of a measurement statement might be: "The dependent variable is the occurrence of a flu vaccine in the 6 months following the intervention, and it is reported as a percentage of the total patients in each group (intervention vs. comparison, which is the independent variable)."

Once the outcome and measurement statements are determined, the next step necessary for executing the measure is to write the formula for calculating that measure. In this instance the formulas would look like this:

TABLE 4.4   Example of Outcome Variable Information

Variable Name	Brief Description	Data Source	Possible Range of Values	Level of Measurement	Time Frame for Collection	Statistical Test
fluvaccdate	Date of flu vaccine administration	Clinic medical records	9/1/2011–2/28/2011 or null for no vaccine administered	Date field	Collected retrospectively in March 2013	N/A
daystofluvacc	Number of days from intervention to administration of flu vaccine	Calculated field using fluvaccdate and intervention date of 9/1/2011	0–183	Ratio	Calculated when all data collected	N/A
Fluvaccin6mo	Indicator of whether flu vaccine was administered within 6 months of intervention	Calculated field using daystofluvacc variable	1 = yes 0 = no	Dichotomous	Calculated when all data collected	Chi-square test of proportions

N/A, not applicable.

Number of patients in intervention group receiving
the flu vaccine in 6-month period

Number of patients in the intervention group

Number of patients in comparison group receiving
the flu vaccine in 6-month period

Number of patients in the comparison group

The next step in the outcomes-measurement plan is to write the details about the necessary variables. Particulars about the variables are similar to those written about the descriptive variable information; in this section it is essential to decide which statistical test to use to measure this outcome. Table 4.4 shows an example of outcome variable information with selection of a statistical test.

Because the focus of this discussion has been on the description of the population or evaluation of successful attainment of the project aims, the decision about statistical testing is limited to tests using one independent and one dependent variable. Multivariate statistical tests and their use are explained in Chapter 8.

SUMMARY

Creating the data analysis plan is a critical step in any project that requires analysis of data. It is created during the overall project-planning stage before implementation begins. A high-caliber analytic plan and its implementation provide DNPs and other key stakeholders and decision makers with the information necessary to make judgments about the value and continuance of each evidence-based intervention or feasibility exploration.

REFERENCES

Ishani, A., Greer, N., Taylor, B. C., Kubes, L., Cole, P., Atwood, M., . . . Ercan-Fang, N. (2011). Effect of nurse case management compared with usual care on controlling cardiovascular risk factors in patients with diabetes. *Diabetes Care, 34*(8), 1689–1694.

Lenth, R. V. (2006–2009). Russ Lenth power and sample size calculator [Computer software]. Java Applets for Power and Sample Size. Retrieved June 12, 2013, from http://www.stat.uiowa.edu/~rlenth/Power

Ovretveit, J., & Gustafson, D. (2002). Evaluation of quality improvement programmes. *Quality and Safety in Health Care, 11*(3), 270–275.

Polit, D. F., & Beck, C. T. (2012). *Generating and assessing evidence for nursing practice* (9th ed.). Philadelphia, PA: Lippincott Williams & Wilkins.

Sylvia, M. L., Griswold, M., Dunbar, L., Boyd, C. M., Park, M., & Boult, C. (2008). Guided care: Cost and utilization outcomes in a pilot study. *Disease Management, 11*(1), 29–36.

Welch, G., Garb, J., Zagarins, S., Lendel, I., & Gabbay, R. (2010). Nurse diabetes case management interventions and blood glucose control: Results of a meta-analysis. *Diabetes Research and Clinical Practice, 88*(1), 1–6.

CASE STUDY

CASE STUDY EXAMPLE: COMPLETE EVALUATION PLAN

Population Description

Project purpose	The purpose of this quality-improvement project is to improve the health status and the efficiency of health care resource use in older community-dwelling patients with diabetes who are receiving intensive care management services.
Name of the population	Older community-dwelling patients with diabetes
Subgroup receiving intervention	Patients with diabetes receive the intervention if they live in geographic region A.
Subgroup used for comparison	Patients with diabetes are assigned to the comparison group if they live in geographic region B.
Source(s) of data	Health plan administrative claims data
Number expected	200 members in each group (based on power analysis)
Criteria for inclusion	Must be enrolled in the Care1 health insurance plan; must have diagnosis of diabetes present in administrative health claims data (defined by presence of two diagnosis codes occurring in same year); must be 65 years of age and over
Criteria for exclusion	Diagnosis of end-stage renal disease; currently scheduled for organ transplant; active cancer treatment
Time frame	Patients are assessed for inclusion and exclusion criteria and subgroup determination in previous year from start date of intervention.

Descriptive/Demographic Information

Variable Name	Brief Description	Data Source	Possible Range of Values	Level of Measurement	Time Frame for Collection
PatientID	Assigned identification number	Same as health plan identification number	N/A	Text	At onset of intervention
Subgroup	Grouping within the population	Assigned	0 = comparison 1 = intervention	Dichotomous	At onset of intervention
Age	Age at start of intervention calculated from date of birth	Health plan enrollment data	65–104	Continuous	Previous 12 months from start of intervention
Gender	Gender	Health plan enrollment data	1 = female 0 = male	Dichotomous	Previous 12 months from start of intervention
Race	Race	Health plan enrollment data	0 = White 1 = African American/Black 2 = Hispanic	Categorical	Previous 12 months from start of intervention
Morbiditylevel	The level of morbidity based on ACG® methodology. (This is collected because it may explain any unexpected differences in the outcomes measure that are not related to the intervention.)	ACG methodology applied to health plan administrative claims and enrollment data	0 = nonuser 1 = very low 2 = low 3 = moderate 4 = high 5 = very high	Ordinal	Previous 12 months from start of intervention
Chroniccondition	Multiple indicators for other coexisting chronic conditions and diabetes manifestations	ACG methodology applied to health plan administrative claims and enrollment data	0 = condition doesn't exist 1 = condition does exist	Dichotomous	Previous 12 months from start of intervention

ACG, Adjusted Clinical Groups; N/A, not applicable.

OUTCOMES, MEASURES, CALCULATIONS, AND VARIABLES

Aim 1

Older patients with diabetes to achieve and maintain appropriate control of their blood glucose levels.

Outcome 1a: The intervention group has a lower mean hemoglobin A1C (HbA1C) postintervention value when matched against the comparison group. Based on evidence from a pilot study at this intervention site and considering corroboration from the literature, the expected difference in mean HbA1C levels is approximately 0.9 (Ishani et al., 2011; Welch, Garb, Zagarins, Lendel, & Gabbay, 2010).

Measure 1a: The dependent variable is posthba1c, which is the name of the variable representing the post value for HbA1C. (Note: If there is more than one HbA1C value per patient in the postperiod, the last value recorded in the period will be used.) The independent variable is the receipt of the intervention, which is represented by the subgrouping variable in the population (intervention/comparison).

$$\textit{Calculation of measure 1a:} \quad \frac{\substack{\text{Sum of HbA1C values in intervention group} \\ \text{6 months postintervention}}}{N \text{ of patients in intervention group}}$$

$$\frac{\substack{\text{Sum of HbA1C values in comparison group} \\ \text{6 months postintervention}}}{N \text{ of patients in comparison group}}$$

Outcome 1b: The intervention group has a larger mean lowering of HbA1C values from preintervention to postintervention when equated with the comparison group. Based on clinical experience, the expected difference in mean lowering between both groups is approximately 25%. (For example, if the mean difference in pre- to post-HbA1C is 1.0 in the intervention group and the mean difference in pre- to post-HbA1C is .75 in the comparison group, the difference in mean lowering is 25%.)

Measure 1b: The dependent variable is the difference in HbA1C value determined at the start of the intervention compared to the value 6 months postintervention. (Note: If there is more than one HbA1C value per patient in a period, the last value recorded in the period will be used.) This is measured as a sum of the postvalue minus the prevalue for each individual patient, and a negative number indicates a lowering from prevalue to postvalue. This variable is named "diffhba1c." The independent variable is the receipt of the intervention, which is represented by the subgrouping variable in the population (intervention/comparison).

$$\textit{Calculation of measure 1b:} \quad \frac{\substack{\text{Sum of the pre/post-differences in HbA1C} \\ \text{values in intervention group}}}{N \text{ of patients in intervention group}}$$

$$\frac{\substack{\text{Sum of the pre/post-differences in HbA1C} \\ \text{values in comparison group}}}{N \text{ of patients in comparison group}}$$

Variables Used for Aim 1

Variable Name	Brief Description	Data Source	Possible Range of Values	Level of Measurement	Time Frame for Collection	Statistical Test
Subgroup	Grouping within the population	Assigned	0 = comparison 1 = intervention	Dichotomous	At onset of intervention	N/A
Prehba1c	Value of HbA1C at start of intervention. This value represents the preintervention value.	Lab submits value of HbA1C to clinic. It is entered in medical record. Clinic submits data set of values for measurement of this aim.	6.0–18.0	Continuous	At onset of intervention	N/A
Posthba1c	Value of HbA1C at 6 months following start of intervention. This value represents the postintervention value.	Lab submits value of HbA1C to clinic. It is entered in medical record. Clinic submits data set of values for measurement of this aim.	6.0–18.0	Continuous	6 months postintervention	Independent t-test used to test differences between intervention and comparison groups for outcome 1a.
Diffhba1c	Difference between HbA1C value preintervention and postintervention	Calculated as postvalue minus prevalue	−12.0–+12.0	Continuous	Calculated when all data have been collected	Independent t-test used to test differences between intervention and comparison groups for outcome 1b.

HbA1C, hemoglobin A1C; N/A, not applicable.

OUTCOMES, MEASURES, CALCULATIONS, AND VARIABLES

Aim 2

Senior patients with diabetes to experience efficient use of health care services.

Outcome 2a: The intervention group has lower mean inpatient hospitalizations postintervention compared to the comparison group. Based on available evidence and clinical experience, the expected difference in means is at least .20 admissions per patient (Sylvia et al., 2008).

Measure 2a: The dependent variable is the count of inpatient hospitalizations between the start of the intervention and 1 year postintervention. The independent variable is the receipt of the intervention, which is represented by the subgrouping variable in the population (intervention/comparison).

Calculation of measure 2a:
$$\frac{\text{Sum of inpatient hospitalizations in intervention group postintervention}}{N \text{ of patients in intervention group}}$$

$$\frac{\text{Sum of inpatient hospitalizations in comparison group postintervention}}{N \text{ of patients in comparison group}}$$

Outcome 2b: The intervention group has a lower percentage of patients with any hospitalization in the postperiod when matched against the comparison group. Based on limited available evidence and clinical experience, the difference in percentages is expected to be approximately 50% (e.g., 10% with admissions in the intervention group and 20% with admissions in the comparison group).

Measure 2b: The dependent variable is the occurrence of at least one hospitalization in the year following the start of the intervention. The independent variable is the receipt of the intervention, which is represented by the subgrouping variable in the population (intervention/comparison).

Calculation of measure 2b:
$$\frac{\text{Count of the patients in the intervention group with an admission in the postperiod}}{N \text{ of patients in intervention group}}$$

$$\frac{\text{Count of the patients in the comparison group with an admission in the postperiod}}{N \text{ of patients in comparison group}}$$

Outcome 2c: The intervention group has a larger mean lowering of inpatient admissions from preintervention to postintervention when equated with the comparison group. Based on clinical experience, the difference in mean lowering between both groups is at least 50%. (To illustrate, if the mean difference in preadmissions to postadmissions is .20 per patient in the intervention group and the mean difference in preadmissions to postadmissions is .10 per patient in the comparison group, the difference in mean lowering is 50%.)

Variables Used for Aim 2

Variable Name	Brief Description	Data Source	Possible Range of Values	Level of Measurement	Time Frame for Collection	Statistical Test
Subgroup	Grouping within the population	Assigned	0 = comparison 1 = intervention	Dichotomous	At onset of intervention	N/A
Preadmcount	Count of inpatient admissions in year prior to start of intervention. This value represents the preintervention value.	Admissions are counted using administrative health plan data.	0–20	Continuous	At onset of intervention	N/A
Postadmcount	Count of inpatient admissions in year following the start of intervention. This value represents the postintervention value.	Admissions are counted using administrative health plan data.	0–20	Continuous	1 year postintervention	Independent t-test used to test differences between intervention and comparison groups for outcome 2a.
Postadmit	Indicator of whether an inpatient admission occurred in the postperiod	Calculated from postadmcount variable (0 indicates no admission; all other values indicate the occurrence of an admission)	0 = no admission 1 = admission	Dichotomous	Calculated when all data have been collected	Chi-square test used to test differences between intervention and comparison groups for outcome 2b.
Diffadm	Difference between count of inpatient preadmissions and postadmissions	Calculated as postvalue minus prevalue	−20.0 – +20.0	Continuous	Calculated when all data have been collected	Independent t-test used to test differences between intervention and comparison groups for outcome 2c.

N/A, not applicable.

Measure 2c: The dependent variable is the difference in inpatient hospital admissions determined by counting admissions in the year preintervention matched against the value 1 year postintervention. This is measured as a sum of the postnumber of admissions minus the prenumber of admissions for each individual patient, and a negative number indicates a lowering from preadmissions to postadmissions. The independent variable is the receipt of the intervention, which is represented by the subgrouping variable in the population (intervention/comparison).

Calculation of measure 2c:
$$\frac{\text{Sum of the pre/post-differences in number of inpatient admissions in intervention group}}{N \text{ of patients in intervention group}}$$

$$\frac{\text{Sum of the pre/post-differences in number of inpatient admissions in comparison group}}{N \text{ of patients in comparison group}}$$

Event Description

Project purpose	The purpose of this quality-improvement project is to improve the health status and the efficiency of health care resource use in senior community-dwelling patients with diabetes who are receiving intensive care management services. As part of this project, all patients with diabetes were introduced to a statewide initiative to reduce readmission rates. This portion of the data plan explores the effects of that initiative on all patients, enrolled in the Care1 health insurance plan, over the age of 50 and with diabetes.
Name of the event	Inpatient admissions
Events exposed to program intervention	Admissions for community-dwelling patients with diabetes who are enrolled in Care1 health plan for 1 full year following the implementation of the readmissions prevention initiative
Events for comparison	None, this is descriptive and compared to a benchmark rate.
Source(s) of data	Admissions are determined from administrative health care claims data.
Number expected	This is estimated at approximately 3,500 patients.
Criteria for inclusion	Any admission for a patient with diabetes in the community-dwelling population. The admission must occur within 1 year postreadmissions reduction initiative. The patient criteria for including admissions are: ■ 50 years of age or older ■ Diabetes diagnosis present in administrative health claims data (defined by presence of two diagnosis codes occurring in the previous year) ■ Must be continuously enrolled in Care1 health plan for 1 year postinitiative start date ■ Community dwelling determined by administrative claims data, excluding anyone with skilled nursing facility admissions during either the preperiod or postperiod
Criteria for exclusion	Any admission to a skilled nursing or rehabilitation facility
Any special populations to consider in measurement?	Yes, patient ID; hospital of admission
Time frame	Admissions measured in the year postinitiative, and all data collection takes place monthly for 13 months postinitiative

Descriptive Information for Inpatient Admission Events

Variable Name	Brief Description	Data Source	Possible Range of Values	Level of Measurement	Time Frame for Collection
Admitid	Identification number assigned to each admission	Assigned	N/A	Text	At end of initiative
Patientid	Assigned identification number	Same as health plan identification number	N/A	Text	At end of initiative
Age	Patient age at admission	Health plan administrative claims data	50–114	Continuous	At end of initiative
Gender	Patient gender	Health plan administrative claims data	Male/female	Dichotomous	At end of initiative
DRGcode	Diagnosis-related group code—a code for the diagnosis related to the admission	Health plan administrative claims data	000–999	Nominal	At end of initiative
DRGdesc	Diagnosis-related group—a description of the diagnosis related to the admission	Health plan administrative claims data	Description related to code	Nominal	At end of initiative
BedType	Description of specialty of type of hospital unit in which patient admission occurred	Health plan administrative claims data	"Acute Rehab," "Intensive Care Unit," "Medical," "Obstetrics," "Psychiatric," "Subacute," "Other"	Nominal	At end of initiative
AdmitDate	Date of admission	Health plan administrative claims data	1–12	Continuous	At end of initiative
DischargeDate	Date of discharge	Health plan administrative claims data	1–31	Continuous	At end of initiative
TotalDays	Total days admitted	Health plan administrative claims data	1–365	Continuous	At end of initiative
Dayssinceprevadm	Number of days between admissions	Calculated from health plan administrative data; discharge day/month of current admission minus admission day/month of subsequent admission	Null, 1–365	Continuous	At end of initiative

N/A, not applicable.

Aim 3

All Care1 health plan older patients with diabetes to experience efficient use of health care services.

Outcome 3a: Care1 health plan patients with diabetes have less than a 15% rate of 30-day readmissions in the postperiod, based on published local benchmark data.

Measure 3a: The dependent variable is the occurrence of a readmission. The independent variable is exposure to the readmissions initiative; however, this cannot be represented in a grouping variable because there is no available comparison group. Therefore, the observed percentage is compared to the benchmark of 15%.

$$\text{Calculation of measure 3a:} \quad \frac{\text{Count of 30-day readmissions in the postperiod}}{\substack{N \text{ of admissions for Care1 health plan older} \\ \text{patients with diabetes in the postperiod}}}$$

Variables Used for Aim 3

Variable Name	Brief Description	Data Source	Possible Range of Values	Level of Measurement	Time Frame for Collection	Statistical Test
Readmission	Indicator of 30-day readmission	Calculated from days from prevadm, and a value of 30 or less indicates a 30-day readmission. The subsequent admission is identified as the readmission yes or no.	0 = no 1 = yes	Dichotomous	At end of initiative	Descriptive

CASE STUDY EXAMPLE: POWER ANALYSIS

In order to decide on the sample size necessary for this project to achieve statistical power, the aims and outcomes from which the determination is made need to be chosen. For this project, it is most important to impact the quality measure of HbA1C and health care utilization, specifically admissions. In examining the sample size necessary for each of these areas, the following aims and outcomes are used, and the next section details the inputs used and sample size required under each scenario.

Aim 1

Older patients with diabetes to achieve and maintain appropriate control of their blood glucose levels.

Outcome 1a: The intervention group has a lower mean HbA1C postintervention value compared to the comparison group. Based on evidence from a pilot study at this intervention site and considering documentation from the literature, the expected difference in mean HbA1C levels is approximately 0.9 and the estimated standard deviation is 1.5 (Ishani et al., 2011; Welch et al., 2010). The inputs for this power analysis are:

Alpha: equals 0.05

Power: equals 0.80 (Remember, this calculator uses an approximation of power to give a rounded whole number for sample size, so this can range between 0.79 and 0.81. It is always best to use the value greater than and closest to 0.80 that gives a rounded whole-number sample size.)

Standard deviation or sigma: This is the estimated standard deviation for the intervention group and the comparison group. For these inputs it is assumed that the intervention group and the comparison group have the same standard deviation and it is equal to 1.5.

Difference in means: This is the expected difference in mean HbA1C between the intervention group and comparison group and is equal to 0.9.

Based on aim 1, outcome 1a, and using the listed inputs, in order to have enough power to detect a statistically significant difference in mean HbA1C levels between the intervention and comparison groups, 45 patients are required in each of the groups (intervention and comparison) (Figure 4.1).

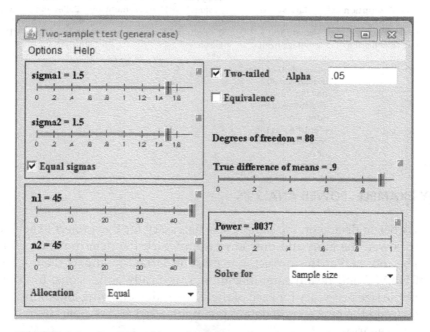

FIGURE 4.1 Sample size calculation for outcome 1a using sample size calculator.

Output obtained using Lenth (2006–2009).

Aim 2

Older patients with diabetes to experience efficient use of health care services.

Outcome 2a: The intervention group has lower mean inpatient hospitalizations postintervention when matched against the comparison group. Based on available evidence and clinical experience, the difference in means should be at least .20 admissions per patient. The literature for this measure shows that the expected standard deviation in a group of similar patients for mean number of admissions is 0.8 (Sylvia et al., 2008).

The inputs for this power analysis are:

Alpha: equals 0.05

Power: equals 0.80 (Remember, this calculator uses an approximation of power to give a rounded whole number for sample size, so this can range between 0.79 and 0.81. It is always best to use the value greater than and closest to 0.80 that gives a rounded whole-number sample size.)

Standard deviation or sigma: This is the estimated standard deviation for the intervention group and the comparison group. For these inputs it is assumed that the intervention group and the comparison group have the same standard deviation and it is equal to 0.8.

Difference in means: This is the expected difference in mean admissions between the intervention group and comparison group and is equal to .20.

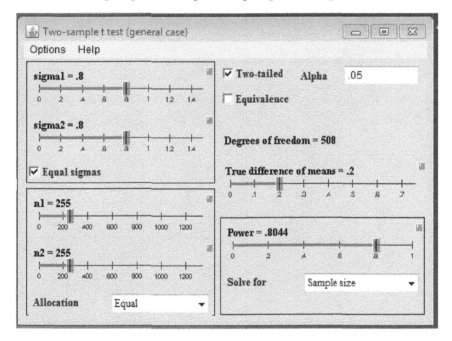

FIGURE 4.2   Sample size calculation for outcome 2a using sample size calculator.

Output obtained using Lenth (2006–2009).

Based on aim 2, outcome 2a, and using the listed inputs, in order to have enough power to detect a statistically significant difference in mean hospitalizations between the intervention and comparison groups, 255 patients are required in each of the groups (intervention and comparison) (Figure 4.2).

In summary, detecting a statistically significant difference in the HbA1C mean (aim 1, outcome 1a) requires a sample size of 45 in each group. In order to detect a statistically significant difference in mean admissions (aim 2, outcome 2a), a sample size of 255 is needed in each group. The constraints of this project are such that the maximum expected amount of patients in each group is no greater than 200. Consequently, the project sample size is high enough to detect a statistically significant difference in the mean HbA1C between groups but likely not powered to detect a statistically significant difference in the mean number of admissions between groups.

CHAPTER 5

Data Governance and Stewardship

MARTHA L. SYLVIA

MARY F. TERHAAR

With the increase in health care data availability, data governance is emerging as a new discipline that focuses on the management of data in terms of risk management, access, terms of use, business processes, definitions, and integrity. Data governance refers to the structure and processes within which stewardship of data takes place (Rosenbaum, 2010).

Doctors of Nursing Practice (DNPs) have responsibilities both as stewards of data managed for the implementation of DNP projects, as well as stewards of data within the entire organizations in which they lead. DNPs have a vital role in setting data governance structures for both purposes. Translation projects that DNPs conduct use data to identify and evaluate the status of important problems and determine outcomes of evidence-based interventions. Because data governance and stewardship structures vary within organizations, it is likely that at some point the DNP may use data sources not already governed by any type of structure or stewardship. It is helpful to understand concepts and duties of data governance and to implement and then follow them when they are not already in place.

LEARNING OBJECTIVES

After reading this chapter, the DNP should be able to:

- Describe data governance and stewardship concepts
- Identify the historical and regulatory context of governance and stewardship
- Recognize basic ethical principles fundamental to data governance and stewardship
- Contrast human subjects research (HSR) and quality improvement (QI)
- Assess data governance processes and practices of an organization
- Develop data management plans suitable for institutional review board (IRB) approval

BACKGROUND

Definitions

Data governance is the term used to describe "a process by which responsibilities of data stewardship are conceptualized and carried out" (Rosenbaum, 2010). Organizations establish policies for access, management, and permissible uses of data; define data stewardship procedures; and determine who can access data and under what conditions they are allowed access.

Data stewardship encompasses the entire process used by designated accountable data managers to carry out a fiduciary responsibility to manage the collection, storage, level of identification, aggregation, procedures for knowledgeable and appropriate use, and release of data (National Committee on Vital and Health Statistics, 2009). Data governance usually also includes a component of ensuring data quality (e.g., whereby common definitions of data elements are developed, vetted, and implemented, or data integrity is examined prior to dissemination). The application of each of the content areas of data governance and stewardship varies across organizations. Generally, these definitions help to form a basic structure.

HISTORICAL CONTEXT OF DATA GOVERNANCE AND STEWARDSHIP

Governance of health care data in the United States is rooted in laws relevant to research involving human subjects; in regulations of data management in health care organizations; and in the history of policies governing data quality, usability, definitions, and accessibility. All of these have developed as data have become more plentiful and available in organizations and governmental agencies. Compliance with the spirit and the letter of these laws is the duty of all engaged in research involving human subjects. Although the DNP is engaged primarily in translation and not discovery, all involved in the work of quality improvement, translation, and evaluation need to assure the same protections to participants as those provided to subjects in research. Moreover, regardless of the focus of the work (on either discovery or translation), nurses as professionals are obligated to advocate for individuals, to protect confidentiality, to accomplish good for those with whom they interact (beneficence), and to do no harm (nonmalfeasance) as articulated in the *Code of Ethics for Nurses* (American Nurses Association, 2013).

LAWS RELEVANT TO HUMAN SUBJECTS RESEARCH

Food and Drug Regulations

The history of data governance in the United States as it pertains to the protection of privacy and human subjects comes under a series of laws for which the primary purpose was often something other than strictly the management of data. The first legislation to address the protection of human subjects was the Pure Food and Drug Act of 1906 that prohibited transportation of illegal food and drugs; regulated food and drug labeling; created standards for strength, quality, and purity of drugs; and prohibited harmful additions to or substitutions for food.

Subsequently, in 1938, the Food, Drug, and Cosmetic Act created the Food and Drug Administration (FDA) that enforced the 1906 laws and the expanded regulation to include cosmetics and medical devices, and mandated premarket approval of drugs (U.S. Department of Health and Human Services [DHHS], 2009b).

Nuremberg Code

Although never adopted as U.S. law, the Nuremberg Code (1947) has significantly informed rules issued by the U.S. Department of Health and Human Services (DHHS) to protect human subjects research (HSR). The code resulted from the Doctors' Trial that was one of many Nuremberg Trials that followed World War II (United States Holocaust Memorial Museum, 2013). In this trial, German doctors were accused and found guilty of human experimentation and mass murder through euthanasia. The code is a set of 10 points addressing the ethics of research involving humans. The 10 points stipulate that: (1) voluntary consent of human subjects is imperative; (2) experiments should provide a "good" to society; (3) the design should be based on prior evidence and research; (4) the methods should avoid all unnecessary physical and mental suffering; (5) the experiment should not be conducted if death or disabling injury is expected to occur; (6) the degree of risk should never exceed that determined by the humanitarian purpose of the experiment; (7) proper action should be taken to protect against possibility of injury, disability, or death; (8) only scientifically qualified individuals should conduct experiments; (9) subjects are at liberty to end participation in an experiment; and (10) the scientist in charge should be prepared to stop the experiment at any point (DHHS, n.d.-a).

Declaration of Helsinki

Also guiding U.S. law and following the Nuremberg Code, the Declaration of Helsinki (1964) further developed the 10 principles of the Nuremberg Code and continues to guide the principles of human research ethics today. The declaration was developed by the World Medical Association and has undergone many revisions—the last in 2007. Although developed for physicians, the principles apply to all human subjects researchers. Its tenets are similar to the Nuremberg Code but much more detailed and modernized (Bosnjak, 2001). Several points are pertinent to data governance today:

- The researcher has a duty to protect the life, health, dignity, integrity, right to self-determination, privacy, and confidentiality of research subjects.
- Detailed protocols should contain statements of ethical considerations; information about funding, sponsors, and conflicts of interest; and provisions for managing the situation of subjects who are harmed by participation.
- An ethics committee must approve studies involving human subjects.
- Studies must be constructed by individuals with appropriate scientific training and qualifications.
- Research involving disadvantaged or vulnerable populations is only justified if the research is responsive to the needs of that population.

- Assessment of risks and burdens must take place prior to research, and benefit must outweigh risk.
- Every precaution must be taken to protect the privacy of research subjects and the confidentiality of their personal information, and to minimize the impact of the study on their physical, mental, and social integrity.
- Research studies using identifiable data must normally seek consent for collection, analysis, storage, or reuse of data except in the situation where, as determined by a research ethics committee, consent:
  - would be impossible or impractical, or
  - would pose a threat to validity of the research
- Investigators have a duty to make the results of their research publicly available; are accountable for the completeness and the accuracy of their reports; and are bound to publicly disclose negative and inconclusive as well as positive results (World Medical Association, Inc., 2005).

National Research Service Award Act

The U.S. National Research Service Award Act of 1974 established rules for the protection of human subjects and created the multidisciplinary National Commission for the Protection of Human Subjects of Biomedical and Behavioral Research that was responsible for studying basic underlying ethical principles of HSR; creating guidelines for the selection of subjects and informed consent; and initiating mechanisms for evaluating IRBs of organizations receiving federal grant funds, which was also a new requirement of the law (United States Congress, 1974).

Belmont Report

The Belmont Report followed in 1979. This report summarized the ethical principles developed by the commission to guide the reputable conduct of HSR. These precepts include respect for individuals, autonomy, beneficence, and justice. They provided structure for the first policies for informed consent, assessment of risks and benefits, and selection of subjects. All are still used by IRBs today (DHHS, 1979).

Respect for Persons, within the Belmont Report and the practice of IRBs, refers to the ethical principle that individual autonomy be respected and that persons with diminished autonomy be protected (DHHS, 1979).

Autonomy describes the "personal capacity to consider alternatives, make choices, and act without undue influence or interference of others" (DHHS, 1979).

Beneficence, according to the Belmont Report glossary of terms, is a moral belief that "entails an obligation to protect persons from harm." It can be expressed in two general rules: "do not harm; and protect from harm by maximizing possible benefits and minimizing possible risks of harm" (DHHS, 1979).

Justice, as stated in the Belmont Report, is the basic doctrine that requires "fairness in distribution of burdens and benefits; often expressed in terms of treating persons of similar circumstances or characteristics similarly" (DHHS, 1979).

These and other terms and definitions can be found in the *Institutional Review Board Guidebook* glossary associated with the Belmont Report (DHHS, 1979).

Common Rule

In 1981 the Common Rule, part of the Code of Federal Regulations (CFR), a federal policy regarding human subjects' protection, established the structure, guiding principles, and oversight of IRBs. The CFR requires additional protection for vulnerable groups, including pregnant women, in vitro fertilization, fetuses and neonates, prisoners, and children (DHHS, 2009a).

REGULATION OF DATA MANAGEMENT IN HEALTH CARE ORGANIZATIONS

In addition to laws governing research of human subjects and use of their data, the laws that apply to health care organizations in managing the data for patients also inform data governance policy.

Health Insurance Portability and Accountability Act

The Privacy Rule of the 1996 Health Insurance Portability and Accountability Act (HIPAA) provided the first comprehensive federal protection for the privacy of health information (National Institutes of Health, 2007). The Privacy Rule addressed both use and disclosure of individuals' health information by health care organizations. HIPAA set standards for individuals' rights to understand and control how their health information is used, although allowing the flow of information needed to provide and promote high-quality health care. This regulation applies to health plans, health care providers, health care clearinghouses, and any other health care organization that transmits health information in electronic form, and protects all individually identifiable health information or protected health information (PHI; DHHS, 2003b, 2003c).

Under the Privacy Rule, covered entities are permitted to use and disclose PHI without an individual's authorization for specific reasons. These include:

- To the individual upon request
- For treatment, payment, and health care operations
- To confirm information with an individual
- For incidental use and disclosure, as in the case of a mistaken exposure where adequate safeguards are in place to mitigate risk
- For public interest and benefit activities that fall under 12 national priority purposes in the areas of public health, safety, organ donation, essential government functions, and legal/law enforcement
- For research with a waiver of consent approved by an IRB
- For a researcher statement that the use or disclosure of the PHI is to determine study feasibility
- For an investigator declaration that research is on deceased patients
- For use of a limited data set for testing, health care operations, and public health purposes with a data use agreement by the recipient ensuring specific safeguards for the PHI within the limited data set. Under these circumstances, the health care organization is required to keep a record of use and disclosure, and to provide this to the patient upon request (DHHS, 2003b, 2003c).

DATA GOVERNANCE AND ANALYTICS TODAY

Health care organizations are becoming increasingly reliant on analytics to guide complex processes and operations, including billing and financial reporting; quality reporting; care coordination; managing of patients' health trajectories; managing populations of patients; program planning, implementation, and evaluation; QI; and more. Prior to 2005, hospitals, health insurance companies, and managed care organizations were the main types of health care organizations using large amounts of data to direct these operations and functions related to patient management. These organizations were the first to design and implement data governance procedures. However, in many cases, formal data governance programs were lacking.

Data governance has risen as a priority across all levels of health care and health care organizations. Even as the number of entities seeking to use data to inform health and health care decisions increases, so has the number and complexity of data sets recognized as valuable in this process. Historically, clinicians might have queried clinical data sets to evaluate usefulness of therapies across groups by age or gender or race. More recently, insurers and payers look to determine return on investment from various treatment modalities and programs by querying financial, clinical, and patient-satisfaction data. The stakes are higher and so too are the demands for the accuracy, specificity, quality, completeness, and reliability of the data used to inform decisions (Chute, Beck, Fisk, & Mohr, 2010). Data stewardship and data governance are the keys to meeting these demands.

QUALITY IMPROVEMENT (QI)

QI has roots that extend deep into the history of man and medicine. Theories of evolution and Darwinian survival of the fittest lie at the center of today's continuous quality improvement (CQI) and stipulate that organizations learning from their experiences and developing institutional memories that drive improvement have a competitive advantage over those that do not. This advantage promotes survival in an increasingly competitive and selective health care market. That market selects for continuation those entities that learn from error, and hardwire strategies to prevent its repetition. Conversely, the market deselects, or selects for extinction, those institutions that cannot, or do not, learn from error and implement strategies to prevent its reoccurrence (Simpson, 2013).

The Joint Commission has long promoted QI as a critical component of its social contract to improve America's hospitals (The Joint Commission, 2012). Providers of health care services began to disseminate in earnest the work of their own CQI activities soon thereafter, and many more began to develop theories, strategies, and structures to support meaningful improvement (Berwick, 1989; Berwick, Godfrey, & Roessner, 1990). CQI has been recently defined as the "combined, unceasing efforts of everyone—health care professionals, patients, families, researchers, payers, planners, and educators—to make changes that will lead to better patient outcomes (health), better system performance (care), and better professional development (learning)" (Batalden & Davidoff, 2007). In order to be effective and demonstrate its outcomes, the extensive combined efforts of CQI must be predicated upon strong and specific data. Thus, acceleration of CQI activities has introduced data demands that can be satisfied only by robust governance and stewardship. Furthermore, CQI efforts themselves require rigorous evaluation to determine if practice based on evidence improves outcomes, and to evaluate the yield of efforts in terms of three specific targets identified as the *triple aim* (Berwick, Nolan, & Whittington, 2008). The *triple aim* articulates the serious intent to harness efforts across disciplines to improve health, care, and cost. Gains in any one area are insufficient, absent gains in the other areas.

Much progress was made before the millennium in regard to structure, process, and measurement (Blumenthal & Kilo, 1998). Nevertheless, the impact of CQI is constrained by weak methods and soft analytics that limit precision and rigor. For CQI to bring about system-wide change and meaningful impact, the data and analytics must meet industry standards found in research. Data sets need to be clean, complete, and error-free. Sample sizes have to support power of the analysis. Data from operational, financial, clinical, pharmacological, and other data sets need to be linked and accuracy assured. Only after such rigor can be satisfied can CQI achieve widespread adoption of evidence in practice.

These multiple concerns inform the data planning, data gathering, and data management work conducted by the DNP. The data plan provides details to describe the source, level, quality, and instruments used to gather data; it describes the population and sample, sample size, demographics, and any additional measures required for reliable evaluation of the outcome of the translation and QI efforts.

THE ROLE OF THE INSTITUTIONAL REVIEW BOARD (IRB) IN TRANSLATION AND QI

The role of the IRB is to protect the rights of individuals who might select to participate in HSR. The IRB and its members are responsible for assuring that research conducted within their entity does not introduce risk of undue harm, that experimental interventions offer reasonable hope of improved outcomes, that patients are fully and honestly informed about the study, that recruitment is fair and does not disadvantage any population, that anonymity and confidentiality are protected, and that participation is fully voluntary (Emmanuel, Wendler, & Grady, 2000). The duties of the IRB relate explicitly to research, but may impact QI activities when evaluation involves patient data or when potential risk to patients requires deliberate thought (Szanton, Taylor, & Terhaar, 2013).

An IRB takes the following items into consideration when determining whether a QI project may be exempt:

- The intent of the intervention in regard to dissemination of results (generalizable vs. local/organizational)
- The desire to fully implement interventions if successful
- The type of risk patients are expected to incur in the project (e.g., whether the project intervention may introduce some type of unintentional harm or risk that is greater than normal risks inherent in the delivery of health care services)
- The type of data used (de-identified, delimited, or fully identifiable; Szanton et al., 2013)

Because the distinction between HSR and QI can be difficult to discern, the Office of Human Research Protection has developed a set of Frequently Asked Questions to help guide those engaged in QI and members of IRBs in their decisions about need for IRB oversight (DHHS, n.d.-b).

Organization-Specific Data Governance Processes

In addition to laws developed to protect human subjects, data governance is also informed by organizational policies. Ethical principles guiding use of data and protection of human subjects/privacy were introduced in this chapter under the discussion of the Belmont Report. Organizations adopt and uphold policies that assure protection of these basic human rights within the context of HSR and provision of care.

To illustrate, each patient's right to autonomy and self-determination are protected through adoption of an informed consent process. Informed consent assures patients have been made fully aware of the risks and benefits of a particular procedure or treatment, leaving them free to select the treatment option they believe best meets their needs. In the context of HSR, informed consent allows patients full access to the information available and full determination of their own personal course of action. In the context of QI, the organization commits to a course of action that the evidence indicates should improve outcomes for the population served and the organization as a whole.

DATA STEWARDSHIP, GOVERNANCE STRUCTURES, AND PROCESSES WITHIN THE ORGANIZATION

Organizations are bound to protect the privacy of data in the context of a culture accustomed to immediate, on-demand access. At the same time, they are compelled to increase efficiency of problem solving and care management that can certainly be facilitated by interrogating aggregate data. Hence, balancing privacy with transparency and at the same time advancing the rights of the individual and the needs of society are the challenges facing every professional from every discipline engaged in care, quality, and research.

Meaningful Use

Meaningful use, as stated in the Centers for Medicare and Medicaid Services (CMS) Final Rule, refers to the intent to capture and share data, to advance clinical processes, and to improve health care outcomes (Centers for Medicare and Medicaid Services, 2013). Consistent with the goal of meaningful use, organizations have charged teams with making decisions about data to be collected, the procedures and structures to be used to gather data, ownership, access, security, integrity, data elements to be included, and entry and storage issues. The steps taken by these groups have significant influence over the work of analysts, investigators, and those engaged in QI. Several themes pervade further discussions and policies. These include privacy, ownership, and access.

Privacy

Privacy is a long-standing concern in health care and a fundamental right of the individual in society. It is defined in the Belmont Report as having "control over the extent, timing, and circumstances of sharing oneself (physically, behaviorally, or intellectually) with others" (DHHS, 1979). Organizations have a responsibility to protect privacy and are obligated to develop robust security mechanisms and procedures to do so (Rosenbaum, 2010).

Ownership

Ownership is emerging as a complex concern. The language of ownership is not even found in the Belmont Report (1979). In the time of paper records, the one who had the paper was thought to own the data. Now, in times of electronic records and proliferation of data, ownership has evolved. Ownership of data is now thought to lie with the generator of that data (DHHS, 2003a).

Access

Access to data about an individual, belonging to an organization, must comply with the practices established by the organization in its capacity as steward. As mechanisms for access evolve, new processes to assure privacy coevolve, and those engaged in QI and HSR need to accommodate requirements.

PLANNING FOR DATA GOVERNANCE

Planning for data governance and stewardship within a particular organization and with respect to a particular project is most effective if the DNP understands and works within the following structures and procedures.

Level of Patient Identification Within Data Sets

HIPAA established the Privacy Rule that, in addition to other items, defines three different levels of identification of individuals within data sets that are used by IRBs in determining approval for research and QI. *Individually identifiable* data identify an individual person and include health and demographic information, or relate to an individual's physical or mental health or the provision of or payment for health care (DHHS, 2003c). In order to be classified as a *de-identified* data set, the following data must be removed:

- Names
- All geographic subdivisions smaller than a state, including street address, city, county, precinct, zip code, and their equivalent geocodes, except for the initial three digits of a zip code if, according to the current publicly available data from the Bureau of the Census:

  - The geographic units formed by combining all zip codes with the same initial digits contain more than 20,000 people
  - The initial three digits of a zip code for all such geographic units containing 20,000 or fewer people are changed to 000
- All elements of dates (except year) for all dates relating to an individual, including:
  - Birth date
  - Admission date
  - Discharge date
  - Date of death
  - All ages over 89 and all elements of dates (including year) indicative of an age over 89 (older than age 89 can be aggregated into a category of age 90 or older)
- Telephone and fax numbers
- E-mail addresses
- Social Security numbers
- Medical record numbers
- Health plan beneficiary numbers
- Account numbers
- Certificate/license numbers
- Vehicle identifiers, serial numbers, license plate numbers
- Device identifiers and serial numbers
- Web universal resource locators (URLs) and Internet protocol (IP) addresses
- Biometric identifiers
- Address numbers
- Full-face photographic images
- Any other unique identifying number, characteristic, or code (DHHS, 2003b)

The requirements for a *delimited* (also referred to as limited) data set fall between a de-identified and fully identifiable data set. It may contain one or more of the following elements:

- Dates, such as admission, discharge, service, date of birth, and date of death
- City, state, and five-digit or more zip codes
- Age in years, months, days, or hours (DHHS, 2003b)

The Institutional Review Board

The DNP should be prepared to make application to the IRB for translation projects. The following items should be explored prior to applying:

- Reviewing the IRB charge, mission, and procedures
- Determining the IRB chair, meeting times, and other policies and processes
- Estimating whether the work requires full or expedited review
- Deciding upon consulting services during the application preparation

The data analysis plan developed in Chapter 4 contains much of the information necessary for completing the IRB request for approval, including definitions of: populations/events and any subgroupings; inclusion and exclusion criteria; the expected number for each group; and descriptive, demographic, and outcome variables. In addition to these elements, the DNP needs to describe the following operating procedures for the data:

- Data storage and access
- Data protection and security
- Data destruction at the close of the investigation

SUMMARY

As originally defined, data governance is "a process by which responsibilities of data stewardship are conceptualized and carried out" (Rosenbaum, 2010). It is incumbent on the DNP to develop effective networks within systems that assure protection of the rights of all of those who participate in translation and QI activities. Because the demand for robust evaluation is great, the need for responsible data stewardship is also great. Stewardship practices evolve as organizations face new challenges and demands, and DNPs can provide effective leadership in this effort.

REFERENCES

American Nurses Association. (2013). ANA Nursing World. *Code of ethics for nurses.* Retrieved September 16, 2013, from http://www.nursingworld.org/codeofethics

Batalden, P. B., & Davidoff, F. (2007). What is quality improvement and how can it transform healthcare? *BMJ: Quality and Safety, 16,* 2–3.

Berwick, D. M. (1989). Continuous improvement as an ideal in healthcare. *New England Journal of Medicine, 320,* 53–56.

Berwick, D. M., Godfrey, A. B., & Roessner, J. (1990). *Curing healthcare.* San Francisco, CA: Jossey-Bass.

Berwick, D. M., Nolan, T. W., & Whittington, J. (2008). The triple aim: Care, health, and cost. *Health Affairs, 27*(3), 759–769.

Blumenthal, D., & Kilo, C. M. (1998). A report card on continuous quality improvement. *Milbank Quarterly, 76*(4), 625–648.

Bosnjak, S. (2001). The declaration of Helsinki: The cornerstone of research ethics. *Archive of Oncology, 9*(3), 179–184.

Centers for Medicare and Medicaid Services. (2013, August 23). CMS.gov. *Meaningful use.* Retrieved September 23, 2013, from http://www.cms.gov/Regulations-and-Guidance/Legislation/EHRIncentivePrograms/Meaningful_Use.html

Chute, C. G., Beck, S. A., Fisk, T. B., & Mohr, D. N. (2010). The Enterprise Data Trust at Mayo Clinic: A semantically integrated warehouse of biomedical data. *Journal of the American Medical Informatics Association, 17*(2), 131–135.

Emmanuel, E. J., Wendler, D., & Grady, C. (2000). What makes clinical research ethical? *Journal of the American Medical Association, 283*(20), 2701–2711.

National Committee on Vital and Health Statistics, U.S. Department of Health and Human Services. (2009). *Health data stewardship: What, why, who, how?* Retrieved July 8, 2013, from http://www.ncvhs.hhs.gov/090930lt.pdf

National Institutes of Health. (2007, February 2). *HIPAA privacy rule.* Retrieved July 8, 2013, from http://privacyruleandresearch.nih.gov

Rosenbaum, S. (2010). Data governance and stewardship: Designing data stewardship entities and advancing data access. *Health Services Research, 45*(5, Pt. 2), 1442–1455.

Simpson, P. (2013). The Chartered Quality Institute. *The history and tradition of inspection, quality control, and quality assurance up to c. 1970.* Retrieved September 30, 2013, from http://www.thecqi.org/Knowledge-Hub/Knowledge-portal/Concepts-of-quality/History-and-tradition

Szanton, S. L., Taylor, H. A., & Terhaar, M. (2013). Development of an institutional review board preapproval process for Doctor of Nursing Practice students: Process and outcome. *Journal of Nursing Education, 52*(1), 51–55.

The Joint Commission. (2012). *Improving America's hospitals: Annual report on quality and safety.* Retrieved August 23, 2013, from http://www.jointcommission.org/assets/1/18/TJC_Annual_Report_2012.pdf

United States Congress. (1974). National Research Service Award Act of 1974. Public Law 93-348.

United States Holocaust Memorial Museum. (2013, June 10). *Holocaust encyclopedia. The doctors' trial: The medical case of the subsequent Nuremberg proceedings.* Retrieved July 8, 2013, from http://www.ushmm.org/wlc/en/article.php?ModuleId=10007035

U.S. Department of Health and Human Services. (1979). National Commission for the Protection of Human Subjects of Biomedical and Behavioral Research. *The Belmont Report.* Retrieved July 8, 2013, from http://www.hhs.gov/ohrp/humansubjects/guidance/belmont.html

U.S. Department of Health and Human Services. (2003a). Federal Register, Office of the Secretary. *Health insurance reform: Security standards; final rule.* Retrieved September 23, 2013, from http://www.hhs.gov/ocr/privacy/hipaa/administrative/securityrule/securityrulepdf.pdf

U.S. Department of Health and Human Services. (2003b). *Health information privacy training materials. Protected health information.* Retrieved September 23, 2013, from http://www.hhs.gov/ocr/privacy/hipaa/understanding/training/udmn.pdf

U.S. Department of Health and Human Services. (2003c). Office for Civil Rights. *Summary of the HIPAA privacy rule.* Retrieved July 8, 2013, from http://www.hhs.gov/ocr/privacy/hipaa/understanding/summary/

U.S. Department of Health and Human Services. (2009a). *Protection of human subjects.* Retrieved July 8, 2013, from http://www.hhs.gov/ohrp/humansubjects/guidance/45cfr46.html

U.S. Department of Health and Human Services. (2009b). U.S. Food and Drug Administration. *The 1906 Pure Food and Drug Act and its enforcement.* Retrieved June 25, 2013, from http://www.fda.gov/AboutFDA/WhatWeDo/History/Origin/ucm054819.htm

U.S. Department of Health and Human Services. (n.d.-a). HHS.Gov. *The Nuremberg code.* Retrieved July 8, 2013, from http://www.hhs.gov/ohrp/archive/nurcode.html

U.S. Department of Health and Human Services. (n.d.-b). *Quality improvement activities: FAQs.* Retrieved September 30, 2013, from http://answers.hhs.gov/ohrp/categories/1569

World Medical Association, Inc. (2005). *WMA declaration of Helsinki—ethical principles for medical research involving human subjects.* Retrieved July 8, 2013, from http://www.wma.net/en/30publications/10policies/b3

CHAPTER 6

Creating the Analysis Data Set

MARTHA L. SYLVIA

High-quality evaluation results depend on high-quality data. This chapter explains the process of going from initial data collection or from the collection of secondary data to creating a final analysis data set. This procedure includes importing data into statistical software, cleansing the data, manipulating the file and/or data, and creating a final analysis data set and data dictionary. Throughout the entire activity and any ongoing analysis, the doctor of nursing practice (DNP) uses syntax as a method for documenting actions taken on the data and the decision strategy leading to those actions.

LEARNING OBJECTIVES

After reading this chapter, the DNP should be able to:

- Perform a data quality assessment
- Understand and implement methods for addressing data errors
- Apply file and data manipulation techniques
- Develop a final analysis data set and data dictionary
- Document data management processes and decision making

PRELIMINARY DATA PREPARATION

Initial and Interim Data Sets

Frequently, the initial data set will not be the final data set used for the analysis. Preparation in the form of data cleansing or assuring quality of the data; file manipulation (e.g., moving variables and merging data sets); and data manipulation (e.g., creating and calculating new variables) needs to be undertaken to achieve the desired condition for analysis of the data set. Throughout the process of creating the final data set, interim data sets are produced. It is good practice to preserve copies of the initial data set as well as interim data sets by saving them to a secure space where they will not be used. After each save of the data set, a working copy should be created from which further interim data sets are created until eventually the final data set is ready. Saving copies of the data set at intervals allows for backup without needing to go back to original data sources if at any time the working data set is lost or corrupted.

Maintaining Integrity During the Data Collection Process

It is imperative to check data integrity throughout project implementation, when primary data are being collected. Errors in data entry that are discovered early can be immediately remedied; this increases the likelihood of clean, high-quality data at the time of project evaluation. One way to ensure data quality is to set limits on the data entry fields. A possible range of values for a data field as well as the format for the numbers (e.g., number of decimal places, percentages, dollars, etc.) can be set when using Microsoft Access or Excel or configuring existing data collection systems. For instance, a limit can be placed on a field for collecting adult weights so that values can be entered only if they are in the range of 75 lbs. to 800 lbs. and have only one decimal place. Another way to ensure quality is to provide option choices for data field values, wherever possible, in the form of drop-down lists. For example, when entering a patient's pain rating from 1 to 10, a drop-down list would provide the choice of selecting the values of 1 through 10. It is also important to use little or no free text fields for data entry. Free text fields allow for many types of data entry errors.

Data quality can be monitored during the data collection process at multiple points during the project implementation by looking at the distribution of values for each variable. This is more easily accomplished if the data collection software allows for basic exploratory analysis of data fields. Statistical software packages Microsoft Access and Excel provide this functionality. Frequency distributions along with graphic displays in histograms and boxplots easily allow for the determination of missing values, out-of-range values, and erroneous values. The techniques for data cleansing and data manipulation described later in this chapter are helpful during this stage of data quality monitoring.

Importing Data Into the Statistical Software

If the data have been collected outside of the statistical software package, the first step in preparing the analysis data set is to import data into the statistical software package. Most statistical software packages will import data directly from a variety of file types, including but not limited to files with the following extension types: *.xls, *.xlsx, *.xlsm, *.dbf, *.sas7bdat, *.dta, *.txt, *.dat, *.csv, *.por, or *.sav. Database tables can also be added by using what is called open database connectivity (ODBC). Statistical software packages such as IBM SPSS Statistics (SPSS), SAS, and Stata provide a graphic user interface function for importing data files and database tables. Prior to importing into the statistical software the data should be cleaned and formatted as much as possible.

Some items to consider for cleaning prior to import into statistical software include:

- Understanding formats for file types that use delimiters
  - Common file types that use delimiters are *.txt or text files.
  - Delimiters are characters used to distinguish and physically separate every value within the data file. It is important to understand which delimiter is used so that the file is imported properly. Common delimiters include: comma, colon, tab, and space.
  - Column headers are usually in the first (header) line, and each line following the header line is a row of data.
- Understanding formats for columns within spreadsheets
  - Each column or variable should have a set format that matches the type of data. This allows for consistency, especially when manipulating data and making calculations on data values. Some common formats include:
    - *Text* – least restrictive and allows for multiple character types. Text fields do not allow for analytical functions to be performed in statistical software and are usually used for inserting comments or notes.
    - *Number* – a general number field that usually accepts formatting of the number of decimal places. A general number field is better to use than more specified number types such as currency and percentage for importing data into statistical software.
    - *Currency* – a number field that permits commas, the $ symbol, and formatting of the number of decimal places (e.g., $5.65; $10,265.65).
    - *Percentage* – a number field that allows for the % symbol and formatting of the number of decimal places (e.g., 5.6%).
    - *Date* – a format that permits the month, day, and year to be entered in a variety of common structures (e.g., mm/dd/yy; July 24, 2013).
    - *Time* – hours, minutes, and seconds can be entered in a variety of common formats using a 24- or 12-hour clock (e.g., 13:30:44; 1:30 p.m.).
- Ensuring that data are entered in the intended format
  - Although spreadsheet software and databases allow for designated formats, it is possible, for example, to enter text into a number-formatted field. Check that all values are consistent with the desired format.
  - The values in text files do not have designated formats, which makes this check more challenging and better performed in the data cleansing phase of analysis.
- Checking for missing data
  - Whole rows: Occasionally, rows of data are deleted in a spreadsheet but placeholders for that data remain in the spreadsheet. When spreadsheets with placeholders for missing data are imported into statistical software, this can result in multiple rows of missing data being transferred. This is a problem when analyzing the data because any data or analytic procedures performed in the statistical software will treat the missing rows of data as valid observations in the data with missing values for all variables in the data set. Rows of missing data should be deleted either prior to or immediately after import.
  - Missing values: It is helpful to do a first check for missing values prior to importing into statistical software. This can also be checked after import in the data cleansing phase.

To import an Excel or text file in SPSS, select **File → Open → Data**. When importing from Excel, on the file type drop-down menu, choose the Excel file extension that matches your file. Next, select the worksheet to import and indicate whether variable names are in the top row of the spreadsheet. SPSS will import the fields in the same format as in the Excel file. When importing a text file, again select **File →** **Open → Data** and the appropriate text-file extension. At this point SPSS will execute a data import wizard that makes it easy to provide the information necessary to import the text file. When importing a database, it is easiest to use the database wizard by selecting **File → Open → Database** to import one database table or multiple linked database tables. At this point SPSS will execute an open database wizard.

Documenting the Steps of Data Analysis Using Syntax

One of the advantages of using statistical software is that it allows the creation of sequential documentation of each step in the analytical process, beginning with the import of data. This is accomplished in SPSS by using a Syntax file in tandem with the data and output files. The syntax file is a text file that records commands or actions performed on the data along with comments that explain these commands.

BENEFITS OF USING SYNTAX

- *Documentation*: The syntax file automatically documents each step used during data processing.
- *Reproducibility of results*: It is impossible to recreate a point-and-click session! Syntax:
  - Allows the analysis methods of a current project to be applied repeatedly. This is especially helpful if data are acquired in batches at different points in time and preliminary analyses are undertaken.
  - Provides ease in adjusting one part of an analysis without having to adjust and rerun the entire analysis.
  - Enables application of the methodology used in the current project to a future project.
- *Means of communication*
  - Supplies a useful way to communicate with collaborators and stakeholders about the specific steps used to manage and analyze data.
  - Provides a means of communication between you and another analyst who may do data analysis for you.
- *Allows access to all SPSS functionality*: Some advanced analytic functionality in SPSS can only be applied to the data by writing syntax.
- *Automatic processing*: For future reference, syntax files can be automatically run without personal oversight—helpful when analyses involve multiple processes or very large data sets (millions of records).

OPENING A SYNTAX FILE IN SPSS

To create settings in SPSS so that a syntax file opens each time SPSS is open, in the data window in the toolbar, select **Edit → Options → General → Open syntax window at startup → Apply → OK**. It is ideal to keep one syntax file for an entire project or one syntax file per final analysis data set, so that the complete history of the analysis is housed and organized together. A syntax file can also be opened in SPSS in the Data window by clicking **File → New → Syntax**. To open an existing syntax file click **File → Open → Syntax** and choose the desired file.

DOCUMENTING COMMANDS AND COMMENTS IN A SYNTAX FILE IN SPSS

Syntax creation can be accomplished by either using the **Paste button** that exists in most command windows of the SPSS Graphic User Interface (GUI) or by copying the commands that are posted in the Output window when executing a command from the GUI.

To paste commands into the SPSS Output window, use the following steps:

■ Using the GUI menu, select any desired function (the most commonly used are under the Data, Transform, or Analyze menu items) and enter the necessary information.
■ Instead of clicking the **Run** option, click the **Paste** option. The syntax is now in the Syntax window.

To copy commands from the SPSS Output window into the Syntax window, use the following steps:

■ Double click the Log listing (on the left-hand side of the Output window) that contains the command that was executed; select and copy the command.
■ Paste the command in the Syntax window.

It is important to place comments between commands in a syntax file. These comments describe what the commands are doing and summarize the decision process in choosing the particular procedures.

■ Placing comments into a syntax document requires that asterisks be used before the text and after the comment, or that the comment begins with an asterisk and ends with a period. This separates the commands from the comments.
   ■ ********This is a comment in syntax**********
   ■ **This is a comment in syntax.

RUNNING SYNTAX COMMANDS IN SPSS

Once the SPSS command lines have been created in the Syntax Editor window, they can be run all at the same time or in selected components.

■ To run all of the commands in the window: From the menu bar choose **Run → All**. The results will appear in the Output Editor window. (Choose other options under the Run menu item as appropriate.)
■ To run only part of the commands: First highlight the commands you wish to run; choose **Run → Selection** or click on the big green arrow on the toolbar. The results will appear in the Output window.

EXAMPLE OF A SYNTAX FILE

Figure 6.1 shows an example of a portion of a syntax file that was created during the analytic phase of a translational project. In this particular selection, two files with different sets of overlapping patients taken from two diverse information systems are combined to determine duplicate and distinct patients. This was a necessary first step in determining the final population for analysis. In this illustration, it is more important to understand the look and capabilities of syntax as opposed to the specific commands and their functions.

```
1   *The issue that is being addressed in this syntax is that there are two care management systems that house data
2   for patients enrolled in a care management program. The first system is a telemonitoring system (TMED) and the second system is a care management
3   program documentation system (CAREMGMT). In this syntax, the two files will be merged and duplicates will be removed.
4
5   *Import data from TMED, which was previously transferred to an Excel file format.
6   GET DATA /TYPE=XLS
7     /FILE='C:\Documents and Settings\Main\My Documents\Work\Asthmaeval\Tmedexport.xls'
8     /SHEET=name 'Tmed_ExportQry'
9     /CELLRANGE=full
10    /READNAMES=on .
11
12  *Format date fields appropriately so that they are all the same and remove unwanted variables from the data set.
13  FORMATS PendedDate OpenDate CloseDate UnmanagedDate EligStartDate EligEndDate (ADATE10) .
14  DELETE VARIABLES FinMgmtCat CurrentMANbr .
15  EXE .
16
17  *Save the data set as an SPSS data file.
18  SAVE OUTFILE='C:\Documents and Settings\Main\My Documents\Work\Asthmaeval\Tmed.sav'
19    /COMPRESSED.
20
21  *Import data from CAREMGMT, which was previously transferred to an Excel file format.
22  GET DATA /TYPE=XLS
23    /FILE='C:\Documents and Settings\Main\My Documents\Work\Asthmaeval\Caremgmtexport.xls'
24    /SHEET=name 'Caremgmt_ExportQry'
25    /CELLRANGE=full
26    /READNAMES=on .
27
28  *Format date fields appropriately so that they are all the same and remove unwanted variables from the data set.
29  FORMATS PendedDate OpenDate CloseDate UnmanagedDate EligStartDate EligEndDate (ADATE10) .
30  DELETE VARIABLES FinMgmtCat CurrentMANbr .
31  EXE .
32
33  *Save the data set as an SPSS data file.
34  SAVE OUTFILE='C:\Documents and Settings\Main\My Documents\Work\Asthmaeval\Caremgmt.sav'
35    /COMPRESSED.
36
37  *Merge the two files to determine duplicates. In this merge rows are being added so that the variables
38  in each file need to be exactly the same with respect to variable names, formats, type, level of measurement, etc.
39  This is why the step to reformat all of the date variables and remove unwanted variables was taken above.
40
41  *The below command merges the TMED SPSS file with the file in which the analysis is taking place, which is Caremgmt.sav
42  ADD FILES /FILE=*
43    /FILE='C:\Documents and Settings\Main\My Documents\Work\Asthmaeval\Tmed.sav'.
44  EXECUTE.
45
46  *Save the new combined file.
47  SAVE OUTFILE='C:\Documents and Settings\Main\My Documents\Work\Asthmaeval\Combined_caremgmt_tmed.sav'
48    /COMPRESSED.
49
50  * Identify Duplicate Cases in the combined file by determining if the same patient id occurs more than once. This command is pasted
51  from using the command data-->identify duplicate cases in the SPSS graphic user interface.
52  SORT CASES BY patientid(A) .
53  MATCH FILES /FILE = * /BY patientid
54    /FIRST = PrimaryFirst /LAST = PrimaryLast.
55  DO IF (PrimaryFirst).
56  COMPUTE MatchSequence = 1 - PrimaryLast.
57  ELSE.
58  COMPUTE MatchSequence = MatchSequence + 1.
59  END IF.
60  LEAVE MatchSequence.
61  FORMAT MatchSequence (f7).
62  COMPUTE InDupGrp = MatchSequence > 0.
63  SORT CASES InDupGrp(D).
64  MATCH FILES /FILE = * /DROP = PrimaryFirst InDupGrp MatchSequence.
65  VARIABLE LABELS PrimaryLast 'Indicator of each last matching case as Primary' .
66  VALUE LABELS PrimaryLast 0 'Duplicate Case' 1 'Primary Case'.
67  VARIABLE LEVEL PrimaryLast (ORDINAL).
68  FREQUENCIES VARIABLES = PrimaryLast .
69  EXECUTE.
70
71  ************ 15 duplicate cases were identified and removed************
```

FIGURE 6.1   Example of a syntax file.

Output obtained using IBM SPSS (2012).

DATA CLEANSING

Data cleansing is the process of determining errors in the data and making adjustments for or fixing those errors. It can also be referred to as assessing and improving the quality of the data. It is one of the most important procedures of data analysis and, when done well, ensures a high-quality and efficient remaining analytic process. Depending on the source of the data, the cleansing process can take a substantial amount of time and the attention to detail should not be underestimated. There are many types of errors that may be found in the data. Some of the most common are described here.

Common Types of Data Errors and Their Assessment

- *Missing lines of data:* Importing data into SPSS or another statistical software package, rows of data that were deleted prior to import may be read by SPSS as valid rows of data with every field missing. These missing rows of data should be eliminated prior to import.
- *Completeness of variables (are all variables present?):* It is important to check whether all expected variables were imported in the analytic data set when importing data or directly entering data.
- *Duplicate cases:* These can occur when a row of data for an individual or event is entered twice. This is usually apparent by the same event or person identifier occurring twice. Duplicate cases can also occur when there are unique event and person IDs, but a substantial portion of the remaining data elements for the individual row are the same. The second situation is more common with manual data entry (e.g., when entering the same survey responses under two different person identifiers) and requires more clinical judgment about determining a duplicate case.
- *Missing values:* This is the most common area addressed in data cleansing. For each variable, an assessment must be made of the frequency of missing entries and the presumed reason for those missing entries. An assessment must also be made of the missingness among related variables for the same individual or event. To illustrate, when examining survey data, it is important to understand the amount of questions within the survey that have missing values for each individual.
- *Values outside of expected range:* Each variable in the data set other than free-entry text data types should have an expected range of possible values. This range is defined in the data analysis plan. It is vital to reassess at this point whether the ranges expected during the planning phase match the ranges seen on examination of each variable in the data set. If they do not match, a decision must be made to either adjust the expected range or conclude that there are values in the data that are out of range. It is crucial to distinguish between outlier values and values that are outside of the expected range that are not possible. The case of outlier values that are valid is addressed during the exploratory data analysis phase. In the data cleansing phase, values outside of the range *that are not possible values* are identified. For instance, when determining the expected age range for a group of older people, it can be assumed that the highest value in the data

set should not be older than the oldest person in the United States—age 114 (Gerontology Research Group, 2013). In this case, a value of age 150 would be considered an out-of-range value and invalid. However, a value of age 113 may be an outlier in the data set but an authentic value. Furthermore, if a value close to and above age 114 is found (e.g., age 116), it is worth assessing whether that value is truly a valid outlier or bad data.

- *Invalid values:* These are broader than out-of-range values in that they are any erroneous or unexpected value or value type. Some situations that can cause invalid data include typographical errors, different uses of abbreviations, and wrong data types in a field (e.g., text in a number field). It is essential to thoroughly assess the characteristics of invalid values in order to later determine the best way to clean the data. For example, in a field that requires weight in pounds for adults, at first glance an entry of 65 might be considered an out-of-range value. However, further assessment of this entry could reveal that the weight was entered in kilograms instead of pounds and therefore the data can be salvaged.

- *Combinations of values for multiple variables that should not occur:* It is helpful to examine the values on combinations of variables to determine whether conflicting information is present in the data. A simple example uses area code and zip code. A valid and in-range area code is determined to be clean data when assessed on its own; however, when coupled with zip-code data it may be determined that the area code is not plausible given the reported zip code (this example is not applicable to mobile phones).

- *Errors related to data entry constraints:* Sometimes the good intentions of data-entry constraints placed in the data entry phase can cause the entry of inaccurate data. Data entry constraints include restrictions to items on a drop-down list; mandatory-field entry; restricted value types (e.g., formatted numbers with two decimal places); and restricted value ranges. It is critical to assess these types of data fields to determine whether forced options for entry may have resulted in data entry that is not reflective of the actual true value that would have been entered if the restrictions were not placed on the data field. This is difficult to assess but should be considered. Sometimes the best way to do this is through qualitative feedback from those entering the data.

Methods for Assessing Data Cleanliness/Quality

The tools used for assessing data quality are similar to those used in other phases of data analysis. The important difference here is the purpose for using these tools at this point: for a specific and pointed focus on data cleanliness. Statistical and graphical functions that display frequencies of values are helpful in assessing categorical data and some continuous data. Descriptive statistical functions are most useful for continuous data with a large distribution of values.

A simple frequency distribution will usually suffice when assessing categorical data. This can be done in SPSS by clicking **Analyze → Frequencies** and choosing the appropriate variables and options. Table 6.1 displays the frequency distribution for a field in an electronic medical record (EMR) where the clinicians were asked to enter a diagnosis for the patient. The only restriction on the field was that it was formatted as a text-entry field. In this project it was necessary to

TABLE 6.1   SPSS Frequency Distribution for Clinician-Entered Diagnosis Data

Diagnosis	Frequency	Percent	Valid Percent	Cumulative Percent
Valid Acute MI	1	.3	.3	.3
CAD	2	.5	.5	.8
CAD, Angina, Hyperlipids	1	.3	.3	1.1
CAD, CHF, DM	1	.3	.3	1.4
CAD, CHF, HTN, DM	1	.3	.3	1.6
CAD, CVA, HTN	1	.3	.3	1.9
CAD, Diabetes	2	.5	.5	2.5
CAD, DM	7	1.9	1.9	4.4
CAD, DM, HTN	4	1.1	1.1	5.5
CAD, HTN	2	.5	.5	6.0
CAD, HTN, DM	3	.8	.8	6.8
CHF	54	14.8	14.8	21.6
CHF, CAD	7	1.9	1.9	23.6
CHF, CAD, DM	3	.8	.8	24.4
CHF, Diabetes	3	.8	.8	25.2
CHF, DM	31	8.5	8.5	33.7
CHF, DM, CAD	3	.8	.8	34.5
CHF, DM, HTN	8	2.2	2.2	36.7
CHF, HTN	8	2.2	2.2	38.9
CHF/CAD	2	.5	.5	39.5
CHF/Diabetes	9	2.5	2.5	41.9
CHF/DM	2	.5	.5	42.5
DHF	5	1.4	1.4	43.8
Diabetes	33	9.0	9.0	52.9
DIABETES	4	1.1	1.1	54.0
Diabetes 2	3	.8	.8	54.8
Diabetes 2; HTN	2	.5	.5	55.3
DM	11	3.0	3.0	58.4
DM, CAD	16	4.4	4.4	62.7
DM, CAD, HTN	9	2.5	2.5	65.2
DM, CAD, PVD	3	.8	.8	66.0
DM, CHF	10	2.7	2.7	68.8
DM, CHF, CAD	2	.5	.5	69.3

CAD, coronary artery disease; CHF, congestive heart failure; CVA, cerebrovascular accident; DHF, diabetic heart failure; Diabetes 2, type 2 diabetes; DM, diabetes mellitus; HTN, hypertension; MI, myocardial infarction; PVD, peripheral vascular disease.

determine the number of individuals with certain chronic conditions (e.g., diabetes, congestive heart failure, hypertension, etc.). This assessment of the quality of the data for the diagnosis variable reveals that it is not possible to determine the prevalence of certain conditions because each condition is entered in multiple formats (e.g., diabetes is entered as DM [diabetes mellitus], DHF [diabetic heart failure], Diabetes, CHF [congestive heart failure]/Diabetes, DIABETES, Diabetes 2 [type 2 diabetes], etc.) and because multiple diagnosis combinations are entered into the same diagnosis field.

Frequency distributions, descriptive statistics, and graphical representations are all helpful for assessing the quality of continuous data. When the amount of possible values is reasonable, a frequency distribution can be used to

TABLE 6.2   Example of Continuous Data Quality Assessment Using the Descriptives Function in SPSS

	Descriptive Statistics				
	N	Minimum	Maximum	Mean	Std. Deviation
Hemoglobin A1C result	4,239	.00	240.00	7.7614	9.76261
Valid *N* (listwise)	4,239				

N, number; Std., standard.
Output obtained using IBM SPSS (2012).

TABLE 6.3   Example of Continuous Data Quality Assessment Using the Codebook Function in SPSS

	A1C	Value
Standard Attributes	Position	1
	Label	Hemoglobin A1C Result
	Type	Numeric
	Format	F6.2
	Measurement	Scale
	Role	Input
N	Valid	4239
	Missing	0
Central Tendency and Dispersion	Mean	7.7614
	Standard Deviation	9.76261
	Percentile 25	6.1000
	Percentile 50	6.7000
	Percentile 75	7.8000

Output obtained using IBM SPSS (2012).

assess data quality as shown in Table 6.1 (100 or more possible values become too much to assess using a frequency table). Descriptive statistics are also useful. Two ways to do this in SPSS are using the Descriptive Statistics function (**Analyze → Descriptive Statistics → Descriptives**) or the Codebook function (**Analyze → Reports → Codebook**). Tables 6.2 and 6.3 show the output for 4,239 rows of values for the variable hemoglobin A1C (HbA1C).

The assessments of the output from the Descriptives and the Codebook functions reveal that there are no missing values but there are problems with the data. The expected possible range of values is between 4 and 20, and in this output the range is from 0 to 240. However, the tables do not give enough information to fully understand the errors. At this point it is helpful to use some of the graphing options to further assess the issue. Histograms and boxplots are the easiest to use when assessing data quality. During data cleansing, these graphing options are utilized mainly to visualize the values that are out of range. The use of these graphs for exploratory data analysis is explained in more detail in Chapter 7. In SPSS, click on **Graphs → Legacy Dialogues** to create the preferred graph.

The boxplot is the best graphical display to understand the occurrence of values that are out of the expected range. Figure 6.2 shows that there are multiple values above and below the expected possible range of 4 to 20. At this point a decision must be made about how to handle the values for HbA1C that are outside of the expected possible range.

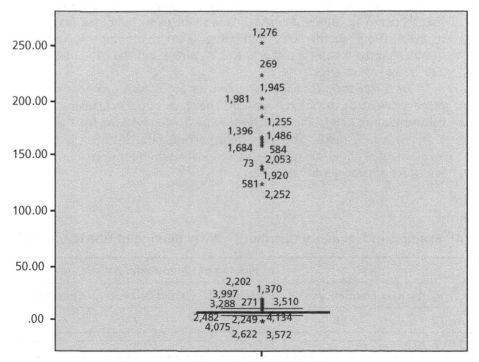

Hemoglobin A1C Result

FIGURE 6.2 Example of continuous data quality assessment using a boxplot graph in SPSS.
Output obtained using IBM SPSS (2012).

A next step would be to determine the amount of values outside of this expected possible range. There are many ways to do this and it is a matter of preference. Some methods include:

- Sort the HbA1C variable in ascending and descending order and count the row numbers that are inside and outside of the range.
- Create a new variable that has a value of 1 when the HbA1C is within range and a value of 0 when the HbA1C is out of range; run frequencies on that new variable.
- Create a new variable that is a binning of the HbA1C value into ordinal categories (e.g., "0.0–3.9"; "4.0–20.0"; etc.) and run frequencies on this new variable. This is the best option because it allows the visualization of values that are close to the expected possible range and far from the expected possible range.

For this example, the HbA1C variable is binned into categories that allow an understanding of which values are closest to and farthest away from the expected possible range. This gives more information about which of the out-of-range values might actually be valid values. In SPSS, one way to do this is by using the **Transform → Recode into Different Variables** option and choosing the old and new variable name and label. In this instance the consecutive five bins, numbered 1 to 5, are created for the new variable with the following labels: (1) "0 to 2.9"; (2) "3.0 to 3.9"; (3) "4.0 to 20.0"; (4) "20.1 to 21.0"; and (5) "21.1 to 240" by using the Range option (under old variable) to define the new variable under the Recode function. Table 6.4 shows the frequency distribution after binning. It is apparent that there are no values of HbA1C close to the expected possible range (no values in the "3.0–3.9" or the "20.1–21.0" ranges). At this point the conclusion can be drawn that the 8 values in the "0 to 2.9" range and the 14 values in the "21.1 to 240" range are in error.

Data cleansing for each variable uses a different process depending on the discoveries made during the session. The steps of data cleansing require analytical thinking in determining each subsequent step and the final point where conclusions can be made. The important part of data cleansing is that a thorough assessment is undertaken that provides justification for decisions made about the handling of poor-quality data.

TABLE 6.4   Example of Frequency Distribution After Binning of HbA1C Values in SPSS

		Binning of Hemoglobin A1C		
	Frequency	**Percent**	**Valid Percent**	**Cumulative Percent**
Valid 0 thru 2.9	8	.2	.2	.2
4.0 thru 20.0	4,217	99.5	99.5	99.7
21.1 thru 240	14	.3	.3	100.0
Total	4,239	100.0	100.0	

Output obtained using IBM SPSS (2012).

Managing Data Errors

ERRORS DUE TO MISSING DATA

In deciding how to proceed with managing missing data, the underlying principle is to ensure that there is nothing about the missing values that would contribute to the determination of the outcomes of the project. To illustrate, in conducting a survey, if a substantial percentage of respondents chose not to answer a certain question, the outcome related to that question could be biased if it were only informed by those who responded to the question. In Chapter 3, an example is described where 40% of the laboratory values are missing for a laboratory outcome for those who received an intervention. In this situation, the reason for the missing data needs to be understood before measuring an outcome using only those with complete data. If there is suspicion that the missing data are enough to bias the results of an outcome, then it may be necessary to forego the measurement of that outcome.

A second principle to consider is that it is important to have each outcome informed by as many observations of values as possible. This means that although a data point may be missing for one variable on one individual row of data, the remaining data for that individual row should be used as much as is possible and reasonable. In the survey example, if one respondent has missed responding to one question, the responses for the other questions should be preserved in the data set. It is rare that an entire row of data needs to be removed from the entire analysis of outcomes.

If the percentage of missing values for a specified outcome is not very high and considered tolerable using clinical and evidence-based judgment, the outcome is usually calculated using those observations for which there is complete data. In the case of missing survey data, most validated survey instruments provide a scoring methodology along with instructions for how to handle missing data. These methods should be used first. Often, when using measures that have a predefined numerator and denominator—as is the case when using measures established by national accrediting bodies such as the National Quality Forum (NQF) and the Agency for Healthcare Research and Quality (AHRQ)—the methods for handling missing data are described in the directions for determining the numerator and denominator.

Another important consideration in handling missing data is in the case of measuring paired observations as in pre/post-testing of knowledge. If the analysis plan calls for paired observations, each observation in the preperiod must match to an observation in the postperiod. If this match cannot be made, each of the observations that do not match needs to be removed from the analysis.

When multiple observations for the same person over time are used for analysis, missing values may be present as time moves forward through the intervention. It is critical to determine whether values are missing because the person is no longer participating or eligible, or because the person is purposely not engaging. For instance, when measuring monthly weight observations for an individual in a weight-loss intervention over the course of a year, if all 12 observations are not present for the person it must be determined whether that individual is no longer eligible for the intervention or is purposely not weighing in. The problem of missing data is not an issue when using longitudinal data that do not have observations linked to each individual over time, as in the case with event data. This is because each measurement point is considered independently from previous measurement points. For example, analyzing all of the admissions that occurred per month to determine the length of stay per admission, each monthly observation of admissions is considered independent of the previous months' admissions.

DETERMINING THE SOURCE OF DATA ENTRY ERROR

If data are suspected or determined to have been entered in error, it is crucial first to determine the nature of the erroneous data. This can be done by communicating back with the source of data entry. It is likely that the source of data entry is either clinical or other staff, the patient, or a monitoring device. If the entry of data is by clinical or other staff, it is helpful to present staff with examples of the suspected errors in the data and solicit feedback as to (a) whether the data are truly in error, and (b) the feasibility of correcting those errors prior to creating a final analysis data set. If feasible, the data should be corrected. When patient data is suspected to have been entered in error, it is difficult to solicit this feedback or to make corrections because patients are usually not accessible during this phase of data analysis.

In the case of monitoring devices (e.g., blood pressure monitoring machines, telemetry, scales, call bell monitoring systems, etc.), it is important to observe the operation of the device and ensure that it is applied correctly and working properly. Historical data captured from a monitoring device may not be able to be corrected, but the device itself should be determined to be in proper working order.

If it is concluded that the errors cannot be fixed, the data should be removed and handled using the methods described for missing data. Regardless of the source of data entry and beyond fixing data errors for the project at hand, action should be taken to change procedures, clarify instructions, fix devices, or do whatever else is necessary so that future data are not entered in error. This is vital for ongoing quality patient care as well as data quality.

FILE AND DATA MANIPULATION

File and data manipulation techniques are useful to understand and apply to initial and interim data sets in order to get to the final analysis data structure. Although it is not always necessary to perform file or data manipulation, the majority of analyses require the use of one or more of these techniques.

File Manipulation

File manipulation consists of maneuvers used to adjust or alter the structure of an entire file as opposed to individual variables. One simple example of file manipulation is a sorting of the entire data set by the order of one or more variables. Other common types of file manipulations and their uses are as follows:

- *Merging data sets:* Data sets can be merged to either add more observations (rows) to an existing data set or to add more variables to a data set.
  - *Adding observations (rows):* This is most often used when the same data structure is captured at different points in time and requires an updating of the data to be inclusive of all observations.

- *Adding variables:* This strategy is commonly utilized when the data for the same observations exist in two different data sets and need to be brought together within one data set for final analysis. For instance, survey data might exist in one data set, whereas demographic data about survey respondents might exist in another data set.
- *Splitting a file:* This type of manipulation splits the file by the values of one or more variables in the data set. Once the file is split, all functions and output are performed separately for each split in the file. This is most often used when the desire is to visualize all output by different groups within the data (e.g., intervention and comparison groups).
- *Aggregating a data set:* This technique aggregates one or more of the variables in the data set to create a new data set that aggregates the values on one or more variables resulting in fewer observations per person. This is most common with longitudinal data sets. For example, aggregation can be used with a data set that has monthly observations of costs per patient to sum each monthly observation into a yearly total (or to pick the highest cost within 12 months or the lowest cost within 12 months, etc.) of costs per patient.
- *Restructuring a data set:* One type of file manipulation under restructuring *flips* a file so that the rows and columns in the original file are reversed, and the rows become columns and the columns become rows. There are multiple options for restructuring a file. This function is useful especially when using secondary data (or survey data from an online survey tool) and the file structure needs to be switched.

In SPSS, these file manipulation techniques are under the **Data** menu item. SPSS does a good job of explaining the use of each function, under the help button for each function, and the information to enter in order to get the desired output data set.

Data Manipulation

Data manipulation is the process of altering existing variables or creating new variables from existing variables. Common data manipulation techniques include:

- *Creation of a new variable from an existing variable:* There are many different ways to create a new variable from an existing variable that allow for a great deal of creativity. SPSS has many options within the graphic-user interface under the **Transform** menu item. Some of the most-used options include:
  - *Compute variable:* This function allows for a direct computation on a variable and provides a wide variety of computation types, as well as the ability to conditionally perform the computation through an *If* statement. A new variable is created that meets the criteria of the computation and any conditional statements. For example, to determine an average monthly cost from total costs for intervention patients, total costs would be divided by 12 and the if statement would be used to indicate that the computation should only be completed if the grouping value is equal to "intervention."
  - *Recode into same or different variables:* This function provides the ability to recode values of one variable into different values on another or the same

variable (it is always better to recode into a different variable and maintain the original variable from which it was created). This function was used in the example earlier in this chapter to clean the HbA1C data.

■ *Date and time calculations:* This set of functions encompasses any calculation that can be done on a date/time variable type. This is most useful when trying to determine the length of time in days, months, or years between two dates. SPSS has created a date/time wizard that can take a user through the steps of any type of date/time calculation.

In SPSS, these data manipulation techniques and many more are under the **Transform** menu item. Again, SPSS does a good job of explaining the use of each function, under the help button for each function, and the information to enter in order to get the desired output data set.

FINAL ANALYSIS DATA SET AND DATA DICTIONARY

The final analysis data set is the one(s) in which the data analysis plan is executed. This is the data set where all of the data have been cleaned and any necessary file or data manipulation has taken place. The final analysis data set should have all of the variables that were described in the data analysis plan and there should be a separate data set for each population or set of events.

The Data Dictionary

A data dictionary is a document that provides descriptive information about each variable in the data set. The information about the variables, with more detail, is similar to the information in the analysis plan. The data dictionary is best created in a table format or in a Microsoft Excel spreadsheet. Common elements of the data dictionary include:

■ Variable name
■ Variable description
■ Data source
■ Variable format
■ Variable measurement type
■ Possible values
■ Coding instructions
■ Coding of missing values

The data dictionary is important because it provides the DNP with a documented history of the data set. It is also essential to use when communicating with other project leaders who may also analyze data. Additionally, it provides a means for interpreting and understanding results in the reporting phase of the analysis. Table 6.5 shows an example of a data dictionary used in a DNP project.

TABLE 6.5   Example of a Data Dictionary

Variable Name	Description	Data Source	Data Format	Measure Type	Possible Values	Coding Instructions	Missing Values
idpatpr	Identification Number	EMR	Numeric 12.0	None	1, 2, . . . ,100	Patient identification number	99
agepr	Age at time of hospitalization	EMR	Numeric 3.0	Continuous	18–115	In years	99
genderpr	Gender	EMR	Numeric 1.0	Categorical	Female, male	0 = female, 1 = male	99
racepr	Race/ethnicity	EMR	Numeric 1.0	Categorical	White, Hispanic, Black, Asian, Native American	0 = White, 1 = Hispanic, 2 = Black, 3 = Asian, 4 = Native American	99
unithospr	Hospital unit type	EMR	Numeric 1.0	Categorical	Medical, surgical	0 = medical, 1 = surgical	99
admdxpre	Admit diagnosis	EMR	String	None	Multiple	—	99
typainpr	Type of pain patient is experiencing	EMR	Numeric 1.0	Categorical	Acute, chronic, acute/chronic	0 = acute, 1 = chronic, 2 = acute and chronic	99
painmepr	Pain medication administered during hospitalization	EMR	Numeric 1.0	Categorical	Opiate, NSAID, other	0 = opiate, 1 = NSAID, 2 = acetaminophen, 3 = other	99
admpr	Number of administrations of pain medication in 24 hours prior to discharge	EMR	Numeric 3.0	Continuous	0–120	—	99

(continued)

TABLE 6.5 Example of a Data Dictionary (*continued*)

Variable Name	Description	Data Source	Data Format	Measure Type	Possible Values	Coding Instructions	Missing Values
lospre	Number of hospital days	EMR	Numeric 3.0	Continuous	1–100	—	99
comnomu	How much comfort did you experience with pain management?	Patient Interview	Numeric 2.0	Ordinal	0–10	0 = no comfort, 1 = 1, 2 = 2, 3 = 3, 4 = 4, 5 = 5, 6 = 6, 7 = 7, 8 = 8, 9 = 9, 10 = great comfort	99
commu	How much comfort did you experience with music therapy?	Patient Interview	Numeric 2.0	Ordinal	0–10	0 = no comfort, 1 = 1, 2 = 2, 3 = 3, 4 = 4, 5 = 5, 6 = 6, 7 = 7, 8 = 8, 9 = 9, 10 = great comfort	99
satcnomu	How satisfied are you with the level of comfort you experience with pain management?	Patient Interview	Numeric 2.0	Ordinal	0–10	0 = not satisfied, 1 = 1, 2 = 2, 3 = 3, 4 = 4, 5 = 5, 6 = 6, 7 = 7, 8 = 8, 9 = 9, 10 = very satisfied	99
satcmu	How satisfied are you with the level of comfort you experience with music therapy?	Patient Interview	Numeric 2.0	Ordinal	0–10	0 = not satisfied, 1 = 1, 2 = 2, 3 = 3, 4 = 4, 5 = 5, 6 = 6, 7 = 7, 8 = 8, 9 = 9, 10 = very satisfied	99
satpmnmu	How satisfied were you with your pain management?	Patient Interview	Numeric 2.0	Ordinal	0–10	0 = not satisfied, 1 = 1, 2 = 2, 3 = 3, 4 = 4, 5 = 5, 6 = 6, 7 = 7, 8 = 8, 9 = 9, 10 = very satisfied	99

satpmmu	How much did music therapy improve your satisfaction with pain management?	Patient Interview	Numeric 2.0	Ordinal	0–10	0 = no improvement, 1 = 1, 2 = 2, 3 = 3, 4 = 4, 5 = 5, 6 = 6, 7 = 7, 8 = 8, 9 = 9, 10 = great improvement	99
satnumu	How satisfied were you with the nurses' efforts to manage your pain?	Patient Interview	Numeric 2.0	Ordinal	0–10	0 = not satisfied, 1 = 1, 2 = 2, 3 = 3, 4 = 4, 5 = 5, 6 = 6, 7 = 7, 8 = 8, 9 = 9, 10 = very satisfied	99
pasvnomu	Patient's self-report of pain severity without music	EMR	Numeric 2.0	Ordinal	0–10	0 = no pain, 1 = 1, 2 = 2, 3 = 3, 4 = 4, 5 = 5, 6 = 6, 7 = 7, 8 = 8, 9 = 9, 10 = worst possible pain	99
pasvmu	Patient's self-report of pain severity with music	EMR	Numeric 2.0	Ordinal	0–10	0 = no pain, 1 = 1, 2 = 2, 3 = 3, 4 = 4, 5 = 5, 6 = 6, 7 = 7, 8 = 8, 9 = 9, 10 = worst possible pain	99
svpatnmu	% of time pain score is ≥ 4 during hospitalization without music	EMR	Numeric 2.0	Ordinal	0–4	0 = 0, 1 = < 25%, 2 = 26%–50%, 3 = 51%–75%, 4 = > 75%	99
svpatmu	% of time pain score is ≥ 4 during hospitalization with music	EMR	Numeric 2.0	Ordinal	0–4	0 = 0, 1 = < 25%, 2 = 26%–50%, 3 = 51%–75%, 4 = > 75%	99

EMR, electronic medical record; NSAID, nonsteroidal anti-inflammatory drug.

Reprinted with permission of Diana Meyer, DNP, RN, FAEN, Director, Center for Nursing Excellence, St. Luke's Health System.
Source: Johns Hopkins University School of Nursing (2012).

SUMMARY

This chapter explains the process of moving from data collection to the creation of a final analysis data set. Syntax is highlighted as a method for documenting the steps of this procedure from importation of the data set into SPSS and throughout the remaining steps of the entire data analysis. The most important goal in creating the final analysis data set is the achievement and maintenance of a high-quality data set in which errors have been identified and managed, and the structure achieves what was outlined in the original data analysis plan. This operation is one of the most time-consuming and possibly cumbersome activities of data management; however, when done well it paves the path to high-quality results.

REFERENCES

Gerontology Research Group. (2013, August 2). *Current validated living supercentenarians.* Retrieved August 5, 2013, from http://www.grg.org/Adams/E.HTM

IBM. (2012). *IBM SPSS Statistics for Windows, version 21.0.* Armonk, NY: Author.

Johns Hopkins University School of Nursing. (2012, August 31). DNP evidence translation project. "No pain provides big gains." *ScienceDaily.* Retrieved August 9, 2013, from http://www.sciencedaily.com/releases/2012/08/120831130653.htm

CASE STUDY

DATA DICTIONARY AND SAMPLE DATA FOR INTENSIVE CARE MANAGEMENT INTERVENTION FINAL ANALYSIS DATA SET

Data Dictionary for Care Management Intervention Final Analysis Data Set

Variable Name	Variable Description	Data Source	Data Format	Measurement Type	Possible Values	Coding Instructions	Missing Values
patientid	Assigned identification number	Same as health plan identification number	String 8.0	Text	N/A	None	Not allowed
subgroup	Grouping within the population	Assigned	Numeric 1.0	Dichotomous	0,1	0 = comparison, 1 = intervention	Not allowed
age	Age at start of intervention	Health plan enrollment data	Numeric 3.0	Continuous	65–115	None	Leave blank
gender	Gender	Health plan enrollment data	Numeric 2.0	Dichotomous	0,1	0 = male, 1 = female	Leave blank
race	Race	Health plan enrollment data	Numeric 2.0	Categorical	0–2	0 = White, 1 = African American/Black, 2 = Hispanic	Leave blank
morbiditylevel	The level of morbidity based on ACG® methodology	ACG methodology applied to health plan administrative claims and enrollment data	Numeric 1.0	Ordinal	0–5	0 = nonuser of health care services, 1 = very low risk, 2 = low risk, 3 = moderate risk, 4 = high risk, 5 = very high risk	Leave blank
adm03	Transplant	ACG methodology applied to health plan administrative claims and enrollment data	Numeric 1.0	Dichotomous	0,1	0 = condition doesn't exist 1 = condition does exist	Leave blank

(continued)

Data Dictionary for Care Management Intervention Final Analysis Data Set (*continued*)

Variable Name	Variable Description	Data Source	Data Format	Measurement Type	Possible Values	Coding Instructions	Missing Values
all20	Asthma	ACG methodology applied to health plan administrative claims and enrollment data	Numeric 1.0	Dichotomous	0,1	0 = condition doesn't exist 1 = condition does exist	Leave blank
car03	Ischemic heart disease (excluding AMI)	ACG methodology applied to health plan administrative claims and enrollment data	Numeric 1.0	Dichotomous	0,1	0 = condition doesn't exist 1 = condition does exist	Leave blank
car05	Congestive heart failure	ACG methodology applied to health plan administrative claims and enrollment data	Numeric 1.0	Dichotomous	0,1	0 = condition doesn't exist 1 = condition does exist	Leave blank
car07	Cardiomyopathy	ACG methodology applied to health plan administrative claims and enrollment data	Numeric 1.0	Dichotomous	0,1	0 = condition doesn't exist 1 = condition does exist	Leave blank
car10	Generalized atherosclerosis	ACG methodology applied to health plan administrative claims and enrollment data	Numeric 1.0	Dichotomous	0,1	0 = condition doesn't exist 1 = condition does exist	Leave blank
car11	Disorders of lipoid metabolism	ACG methodology applied to health plan administrative claims and enrollment data	Numeric 1.0	Dichotomous	0,1	0 = condition doesn't exist 1 = condition does exist	Leave blank
car12	Acute myocardial infarction	ACG methodology applied to health plan administrative claims and enrollment data	Numeric 1.0	Dichotomous	0,1	0 = condition doesn't exist 1 = condition does exist	Leave blank

car13	Cardiac arrest, shock	ACG methodology applied to health plan administrative claims and enrollment data	Numeric 1.0	Dichotomous	0,1	0 = condition doesn't exist 1 = condition does exist	Leave blank
car20	Hypertension	ACG methodology applied to health plan administrative claims and enrollment data	Numeric 1.0	Dichotomous	0,1	0 = condition doesn't exist 1 = condition does exist	Leave blank
end20	Diabetes	ACG methodology applied to health plan administrative claims and enrollment data	Numeric 1.0	Dichotomous	0,1	0 = condition doesn't exist 1 = condition does exist	Leave blank
eye01	Ophthalmic signs and symptoms	ACG methodology applied to health plan administrative claims and enrollment data	Numeric 1.0	Dichotomous	0,1	0 = condition doesn't exist 1 = condition does exist	Leave blank
eye02	Blindness	ACG methodology applied to health plan administrative claims and enrollment data	Numeric 1.0	Dichotomous	0,1	0 = condition doesn't exist 1 = condition does exist	Leave blank
eye08	Glaucoma	ACG methodology applied to health plan administrative claims and enrollment data	Numeric 1.0	Dichotomous	0,1	0 = condition doesn't exist 1 = condition does exist	Leave blank
eye13	Diabetic retinopathy	ACG methodology applied to health plan administrative claims and enrollment data	Numeric 1.0	Dichotomous	0,1	0 = condition doesn't exist 1 = condition does exist	Leave blank
gas05	Chronic liver disease	ACG methodology applied to health plan administrative claims and enrollment data	Numeric 1.0	Dichotomous	0,1	0 = condition doesn't exist 1 = condition does exist	Leave blank

(continued)

Data Dictionary for Care Management Intervention Final Analysis Data Set (*continued*)

Variable Name	Variable Description	Data Source	Data Format	Measurement Type	Possible Values	Coding Instructions	Missing Values
gas12	Chronic pancreatitis	ACG methodology applied to health plan administrative claims and enrollment data	Numeric 1.0	Dichotomous	0,1	0 = condition doesn't exist 1 = condition does exist	Leave blank
mal20	Cancer	ACG methodology applied to health plan administrative claims and enrollment data	Numeric 1.0	Dichotomous	0,1	0 = condition doesn't exist 1 = condition does exist	Leave blank
mus03	Degenerative joint disease	ACG methodology applied to health plan administrative claims and enrollment data	Numeric 1.0	Dichotomous	0,1	0 = condition doesn't exist 1 = condition does exist	Leave blank
nur03	Peripheral neuropathy	ACG methodology applied to health plan administrative claims and enrollment data	Numeric 1.0	Dichotomous	0,1	0 = condition doesn't exist 1 = condition does exist	Leave blank
nur05	Cerebrovascular disease	ACG methodology applied to health plan administrative claims and enrollment data	Numeric 1.0	Dichotomous	0,1	0 = condition doesn't exist 1 = condition does exist	Leave blank
nur06	Parkinson's disease	ACG methodology applied to health plan administrative claims and enrollment data	Numeric 1.0	Dichotomous	0,1	0 = condition doesn't exist 1 = condition does exist	Leave blank
nur11	Dementia and delirium	ACG methodology applied to health plan administrative claims and enrollment data	Numeric 1.0	Dichotomous	0,1	0 = condition doesn't exist 1 = condition does exist	Leave blank

nut03	Obesity	Numeric 1.0	Dichotomous	0,1	0 = condition doesn't exist 1 = condition does exist	Leave blank
psy01	Anxiety, neuroses	Numeric 1.0	Dichotomous	0,1	0 = condition doesn't exist 1 = condition does exist	Leave blank
psy03	Tobacco use	Numeric 1.0	Dichotomous	0,1	0 = condition doesn't exist 1 = condition does exist	Leave blank
psy09	Depression	Numeric 1.0	Dichotomous	0,1	0 = condition doesn't exist 1 = condition does exist	Leave blank
rec03	Chronic ulcer of the skin	Numeric 1.0	Dichotomous	0,1	0 = condition doesn't exist 1 = condition does exist	Leave blank
ren01	Chronic renal failure	Numeric 1.0	Dichotomous	0,1	0 = condition doesn't exist 1 = condition does exist	Leave blank
res04	Emphysema, chronic bronchitis, COPD	Numeric 1.0	Dichotomous	0,1	0 = condition doesn't exist 1 = condition does exist	Leave blank
preadmcount	Count of inpatient admissions in year prior to start of intervention	Numeric 3.0	Ratio	0–20	None	Leave blank

All descriptions for the dichotomous rows: "ACG methodology applied to health plan administrative claims and enrollment data". preadmcount: "Admissions are counted using administrative health plan data."

(continued)

Data Dictionary for Care Management Intervention Final Analysis Data Set (continued)

Variable Name	Variable Description	Data Source	Data Format	Measurement Type	Possible Values	Coding Instructions	Missing Values
postadmcount	Count of inpatient admissions in year following the start of intervention	Admissions are counted using administrative health plan data.	Numeric 3.0	Ratio	0–20	None	Leave blank
postadmit	Indicator of inpatient admission in the postperiod	Calculated from postadmcount variable (0 indicates no admission, all other values indicate the occurrence of an admission)	Numeric 1.0	Dichotomous	0,1	0 = no admission, 1 = admission	Leave blank
diffadm	Difference in post/preadmissions	Calculated as postvalue minus prevalue	Numeric 9.0	Continuous	–20.0– +20.0	None	Leave blank
preHbA1C	Prehemoglobin A1C value	Lab submits value of HbA1C to clinic that is entered in medical record. Clinic submits data set of values for measurement of this aim.	Numeric 4.1	Continuous	6.0–18.0	None	Leave blank
postHbA1C	Posthemoblobin A1C value	Lab submits value of HbA1C to clinic that is entered in medical record. Clinic submits data set of values for measurement of this aim.	Numeric 4.1	Continuous	6.0–18.0	None	Leave blank
diffHbA1C	Difference between count of inpatient preadmissions and postadmissions	Calculated as postvalue minus prevalue	Numeric 4.1	Continuous	-12.0– +12.0	None	Leave blank

ACG, Adjusted Clinical Groups; AMI, acute myocardial infarction; COPD, chronic obstructive pulmonary disease; HbA1C, hemoglobin A1C; N/A, not applicable.

Sample Data for Care Management Intervention Final Analysis Data Set

Patientid	Subgroup	Age	Gender	Race	Morbidity-level	Adm03	All20	Car03	Rec03	Ren01	Res04	Preadm count	Post adm count	Post-admit	Diffadm	Pre HbA1C	Post HbA1C	Diff HbA1C
3	Comparison	76	F	African American/Black	Very high risk	No	No	Yes	No	No	No	0	0	No	0	8.6	7.9	−0.7
12	Comparison	76	F	African American/Black	Very high risk	No	No	Yes	No	Yes	Yes	0	3	yes	3	8.5	10.2	1.7
15	Intervention	76	M	African American/Black	High risk	No	Yes	No	Yes	No	No	0	0	No	0	6	6.5	0.5
17	Intervention	67	M	African American/Black	High risk	No	No	No	No	No	No	0	0	No	0	8.8	7.1	−1.7
18	Intervention	86	M	African American/Black	High risk	No0	No	Yes	No	No	No	0	0	No	0	8.6	8.1	−0.5
23	Intervention	67	F	White	High risk	No	No	No	No	No	No	0	0	No	0	8.2	7.6	−0.6
32	Comparison	80	M	White	Low risk	No	No	No	No	Yes	No	0	0	No	0	9.5	7.7	−1.8
32	Intervention	81	F	African American/Black	Very high risk	No	No	Yes	No	No	No	2	1	Yes	−1	11.1	7.7	−3.4
34	Comparison	74	M	White	High risk	No	No	No	No	No	No	0	3	Yes	3	6.2	11.2	5
41	Intervention	75	F	Hispanic	Moderate risk	No	No	No	No	No	No	0	0	No	0	8.2	7.2	−1

Note: Many condition indicators have been removed to show other data fields.

Readmissions File Creation Using SPSS

The data set that was provided by the health plan is not in the structure that is necessary to calculate the readmissions outcome measure. Therefore, file and data manipulation techniques need to be applied. The following process outlines the steps taken to create the final analysis data set.

1. Original file from the health plan has 4,152 rows (or admissions) and is structured as follows:

Variable Name	Variable Description
AdmitID	Admission ID
PatientID	Patient ID
Age	Patient age
Gender	Patient gender
DRGCode	Diagnostic-related group code
DRGDesc	Diagnostic-related group code description
BedType	Bed-type description
Admmonth	Month of admission
Admday	Day of admission
Dismonth	Month of discharge
Disday	Day of discharge
TotalDays	Total Days for admission

2. A "Year" variable is created by using **Transform → Compute** function and setting year equal to 2013 (all dates are within the same calendar year).
   a. Create "AdmissionDate" and "DischargeDate" variables applying the "Admmonth," "Admday," "Dismonth," "Disday," and "Year" variables. This is done utilizing the **Data → Date and Time Wizard** function using the "Create a date/time variable from variables holding parts of dates or times" option.
   b. The new variables are checked manually by looking at some random cases to ensure the calculation seems correct.
3. Identify any duplicate admission dates by patient using the **Data → Identify Duplicate Cases** function.
   a. Duplicate admissions for 44 patients were identified and all were determined to be 1-day admissions prior to a discharge; therefore, the 1-day admissions were removed and the admissions with the total number of days in each facility/unit were kept.
   b. There are now 4,108 rows in the file.
4. In order to calculate the days between admissions that will allow for a calculation of readmissions within 30 days, the data set needs to be restructured so that all of the data for each patient is on 1 line/row per patient. (The data will later

be restructured back to the original longitudinal form to create the indicator of a readmission.) Prior to any restructuring the data set is saved and stored. Also before restructuring, variables that are not necessary going forward are removed.

   a. The following unneeded variables were removed:
      – admmonth, admday, dismonth, disday, Year

5. The data set is restructured using the following steps:
   a. Select the **Data → Restructure** function to open the **Restructure Data Wizard**.
   b. Use the option to "Restructure selected cases into variables."
   c. The identifier variable is the "PatientID" and an index variable is not necessary.
   d. Choose the option to sort the data.
   e. For the order of new variable groups, choose the option to group by original variable.
   f. For the case count variable, check the option to count the number of cases in the current data used to create a new case. This will provide a count of admissions per patient.

6. The new data set after restructuring contains 14 variables for each variable in the original data set and the new data set has a row for each unique patient. In this example, PatientID and Gender are the only variables that do not vary by patient, so only 1 variable is created for each of these. A total of 14 new variables have been created because the highest number of admissions for any one patient in the data set is 14. Some patients will not have values for all of the 14 new variables created. Patients will only have values for the number of admissions that they had in the original data set (otherwise the value is missing).
   a. The restructured data set has 2,470 rows (individual patients).
   b. Here is the new variable list:

PatientID	Age.1	DRGCode.4	DRGDesc.7	BedType.10	TotalDays.13	Dischargedate.2
Gender	Age.2	DRGCode.5	DRGDesc.8	BedType.11	TotalDays.14	Dischargedate.3
TotalAdmits	Age.3	DRGCode.6	DRGDesc.9	BedType.12	Admitdate.1	Dischargedate.4
AdmitID.1	Age.4	DRGCode.7	DRGDesc.10	BedType.13	Admitdate.2	Dischargedate.5
AdmitID.2	Age.5	DRGCode.8	DRGDesc.11	BedType.14	Admitdate.3	Dischargedate.6
AdmitID.3	Age.6	DRGCode.9	DRGDesc.12	TotalDays.1	Admitdate.4	Dischargedate.7
AdmitID.4	Age.7	DRGCode.10	DRGDesc.13	TotalDays.2	Admitdate.5	Dischargedate.8
AdmitID.5	Age.8	DRGCode.11	DRGDesc.14	TotalDays.3	Admitdate.6	Dischargedate.9
AdmitID.6	Age.9	DRGCode.12	BedType.1	TotalDays.4	Admitdate.7	Dischargedate.10
AdmitID.7	Age.10	DRGCode.13	BedType.2	TotalDays.5	Admitdate.8	Dischargedate.11
AdmitID.8	Age.11	DRGCode.14	BedType.3	TotalDays.6	Admitdate.9	Dischargedate.12
AdmitID.9	Age.12	DRGDesc.1	BedType.4	TotalDays.7	Admitdate.10	Dischargedate.13
AdmitID.10	Age.13	DRGDesc.2	BedType.5	TotalDays.8	Admitdate.11	Dischargedate.14
AdmitID.11	Age.14	DRGDesc.3	BedType.6	TotalDays.9	Admitdate.12	
AdmitID.12	DRGCode.1	DRGDesc.4	BedType.7	TotalDays.10	Admitdate.13	
AdmitID.13	DRGCode.2	DRGDesc.5	BedType.8	TotalDays.11	Admitdate.14	
AdmitID.14	DRGCode.3	DRGDesc.6	BedType.9	TotalDays.12	Dischargedate.1	

7. Next, the number of days between each discharge date and the subsequent admission date is calculated. This is done by using the **Transform → Compute Variable** function as many times as necessary with the following SPSS formulas (note, this can also be done using the Date/Time Wizard in SPSS):
   a. Dayssinceprevadm.2 = DATEDIF (Admitdate.2, Dischargedate.1, "days")
   b. Dayssinceprevadm.3 = DATEDIF (Admitdate.3, Dischargedate.2, "days")
   c. Dayssinceprevadm.4 = DATEDIF (Admitdate.4, Dischargedate.3, "days")
   d. Dayssinceprevadm.5 = DATEDIF (Admitdate.5, Dischargedate.4, "days")
   e. Dayssinceprevadm.6 = DATEDIF (Admitdate.6, Dischargedate.5, "days")
   f. Dayssinceprevadm.7 = DATEDIF (Admitdate.7, Dischargedate.6, "days")
   g. Continue this same pattern of formulas until reaching the last admission—14
   Note that these steps are easier to accomplish by using the **Transform → Compute Variable** function once and pasting the command into the Syntax window. The command can then be copied with the numbers changed as many times as necessary, and the command to create all of the "Dayssinceprevadm" can be run at once. Also note that the variable-naming pattern is similar to that created when restructuring the data file. This is because the data file will be changed back to calculate readmissions.
   h. There is no value for Dayssinceprevadm.1, but the variable is created so that it is in place for the restructuring back to the original form (there needs to be a total of 14 variables for each group that will be restructured back into 1 variable in the original configuration).
      – COMPUTE Dayssinceprevadm.1 = $SYSMIS.
   i. The new variables are checked manually by looking at some random cases to ensure the calculation seems correct.
8. The data set is restructured back using the following steps:
   a. Select the **Data → Restructure** function to open the **Restructure Data Wizard**.
      – Choose the option to restructure selected variables into cases.
   b. Use the option to restructure more than 1 variable, and in this case 9 variables were entered (9 new variables will be created from the variables in the current data set).
   c. Enter each grouping of variables in the current data set that will be restructured into 1 variable in the new data set (total of 9 new variables with 14 variables entered to transform into each: for instance, "admitdate.1" through "admitdate.14" will restructure into the variable "admitdate").
   d. Enter each fixed variable (these are variables for which there is only 1 variable in the current data set: in this case, PatientID, Gender, TotalAdmits).
   e. Choose to create 1 index variable and order index values sequentially (this will produce a variable that allows for ordering of the admissions per patient).
   f. Pick discarding the data of missing or blank values (this is important because all of that data for those who do not have a total of 14 admissions will be cleaned by choosing this option).
   g. Elect to count the new cases created and create a count variable.
9. The new file has the following structure. The Admitnumber and Totaladmits variables were created and renamed during the file restructuring.

Variable Name	Variable Description
AdmitID	Admission ID
PatientID	Patient ID
Age	Patient age
Gender	Patient gender
TotalAdmits	Total number of admissions for patient
DRGCode	Diagnostic-related group code
DRGDesc	Diagnostic-related group code description
BedType	Bed-type description
AdmitNumber	Sequential number of admissions
AdmitDate	Date of current admission
DischargeDate	Date of current discharge
TotalDays	Total number of days for current admission
Dayssinceprevadm	Days since previous admission

10. A variable is next created to indicate whether the current admission is a readmission. This is calculated from the "Dayssinceprevadm" variable. This is accomplished utilizing the following process:
    a. Choose **Transform → Recode Into Different Variables**
    b. Input (old) variable = "Dayssinceprevadm" and output (new) variable = "Readmission" (the label is "indicator of a readmission").
    c. Old value range of "0 through 30" will have a new value of "1."
    d. Old value range of 31 through HIGHEST will have a new value of "0."
    e. Old value of System or user missing will have a new value of System missing.
    Note, the readmissions variable is the key outcome variable for this part of the project. Multiple checks using frequencies with combinations of variables, as well as manually reviewing the data set, are performed to ensure that this variable has been calculated correctly.

DATA DICTIONARY AND SAMPLE DATA FOR READMISSIONS INTERVENTION FINAL ANALYSIS DATA SET

Data Dictionary for Readmissions Intervention Final Analysis Data Set

Variable Name	Variable Description	Data Source	Data Format	Measurement Type	Possible Values	Coding Instructions	Missing Values
AdmitID	Admission ID	Assigned	String 8.0	Text	N/A	None	Not allowed
PatientID	Patient ID	Same as health plan identification number	String 8.0	Text	N/A	None	Not allowed
Age	Patient age at admission	Health plan administrative claims data	Numeric 3.0	Continuous	50–115	None	Leave blank
Gender	Patient gender	Health plan administrative claims data	Numeric 2.0	Dichotomous	0,1	0 = male, 1 = female	Leave blank
TotalAdmits	Total number of admissions for patient	Calculated from health plan administrative claims data	Numeric 4.0	Continuous	0–15	None	Leave blank
DRGCode	Diagnostic-related group code	Health plan administrative claims data	Numeric 3.0	Nominal	1–1,000	None	Leave blank
DRGDesc	Diagnostic-related group code description	Health plan administrative claims data	String 240.0	Text	N/A	None	Leave blank
BedType	Bed-type description	Health plan administrative claims data	String 150.0	Text	N/A	None	Leave blank
AdmitNumber	Sequential number of admissions by patient	Calculated from health plan administrative claims data	Numeric 3.0	Continuous	0–15	None	Leave blank
AdmitDate	Date of current admission	Calculated from health plan administrative claims data	Date 10.0	Date/Time	1/1/2013–12/31/2013	None	Leave blank
DischargeDate	Date of current discharge	Calculated from health plan administrative claims data	Date 10.0	Date/Time	1/1/2013–12/31/2013	None	Leave blank
TotalDays	Total number of days for current admission	Calculated from health plan administrative claims data	Numeric 3.0	Continuous	1–365	None	Leave blank
Dayssinceprevadm	Days since previous admission	Calculated from health plan administrative claims data	Numeric 3.0	Continuous	0–365		Leave blank
Readmission	Indicator of a readmission	Calculated from health plan administrative claims data	Numeric 1.0	Dichotomous	0,1	0 = no admission, 1 = admission	Leave blank

N/A, not applicable.

Sample Data for Readmissions Intervention Final Analysis Data Set

Admit ID	Patient ID	Gender	Total Admits	Age	DRG Code	DRG Desc	Bed Type	Admit Number	Admit Date	Discharge Date	Total Day	Dayssince prevadm	Read-mission
40	1444	F	1	57	691	lymphoma, myeloma & non-acute leukemia	MEDICAL	1	3/12/2013	3/18/2013	6		
135	1203	F	2	58	55	head trauma w/ coma > 1 hr or hemorrhage	INTENSIVE CARE UNIT	1	8/16/2013	8/21/2013	5		
136	1203	F	2	58	55	head trauma w/ coma > 1 hr or hemorrhage	MEDICAL	2	8/23/2013	8/26/2013	3	2	1
301	2360	F	1	55	425	electrolyte disorder except hypovolemia related	MEDICAL	1	12/15/2013	12/29/2013	14		
314	2080	M	1	62	225	appendectomy	MEDICAL	1	8/25/2013	8/27/2013	2		
343	2205	F	1	55	143	other respiratory diagnoses except signs, symptoms, & minor diagnoses	MEDICAL	1	8/31/2013	9/4/2013	4		
428	291	M	1	71	720	septicemia & disseminated infections	MEDICAL	1	4/11/2013	4/12/2013	1		
444	2208	F	1	57	321	cervical spinal fusion & other back/neck procedures except disc excision/ decompression	INTENSIVE CARE UNIT	1	3/17/2013	3/18/2013	1		

Sample Data for Readmissions Intervention Final Analysis Data Set (*continued*)

Admit ID	Patient ID	Gender	Total Admits	Age	DRG Code	DRG Desc	Bed Type	Admit Number	Admit Date	Discharge Date	Total Day	Dayssince prevadm	Read-mission
504	1145	F	1	50	120	major respiratory & chest procedures	MEDICAL	1	11/7/2013	11/10/2013	3		
518	1984	M	1	52	722	fever	MEDICAL	1	12/4/2013	12/6/2013	2		
594	711	M	1	52	253	other & unspecified gastrointestinal hemorrhage	INTENSIVE CARE UNIT	1	7/20/2013	7/22/2013	2		
616	676	M	1	58	314	foot & toe procedures	MEDICAL	1	10/27/2013	10/29/2013	2		
640	108	F	2	58	203	chest pain	MEDICAL	1	4/15/2013	4/17/2013	2		
641	108	F	2	59	121	other respiratory & chest procedures	MEDICAL	2	7/13/2013	7/19/2013	6	87	0
895	308	F	1	58	442	kidney & urinary tract procedures for malignancy	MEDICAL	1	11/28/2013	12/5/2013	8		
1000	1195	F	1	53	302	knee joint replacement	MEDICAL	1	3/17/2013	3/21/2013	4		
1111	1474	M	1	53	142	interstitial lung disease	MEDICAL	1	8/1/2013	8/4/2013	3		
1140	1010	M	1	62	201	cardiac arrhythmia & conduction disorders	MEDICAL	1	6/11/2013	6/15/2013	4		
1304	523	F	1	82	52	nontraumatic stupor & coma	MEDICAL	1	10/27/2013	11/1/2013	5		

(continued)

Sample Data for Readmissions Intervention Final Analysis Data Set (*continued*)

Admit ID	Patient ID	Gender	Total Admits	Age	DRG Code	DRG Desc	Bed Type	Admit Number	Admit Date	Discharge Date	Total Day	Dayssince prevadm	Read-mission
1314	2363	M	1	50	310	intervertebral disc excision & decompression	MEDICAL	1	2/3/2013	2/4/2013	1		
1323	1603	F	1	52	223	other small & large bowel procedures	MEDICAL	1	1/24/2013	1/28/2013	4		
1494	1044	F	2	65	139	other pneumonia	MEDICAL	1	3/31/2013	4/4/2013	4		
1495	1044	F	2	65	425	electrolyte disorders except hypovolemia related	INTENSIVE CARE UNIT	2	4/24/2013	4/25/2013	1	20	1
1534	2131	F	1	56	383	cellulitis & other bacterial skin infections	MEDICAL	1	7/4/2013	7/5/2013	1		
1889	912	F	1	51	139	other pneumonia	MEDICAL	1	12/5/2013	12/9/2013	4		
1905	2229	M	1	58	139	other pneumonia	MEDICAL	1	7/21/2013	7/24/2013	3		
1978	1683	F	5	60	463	kidney & urinary tract infections	MEDICAL	2	10/7/2013	10/8/2013	1	244	0
1979	1683	F	5	60	460	renal failure	MEDICAL	3	11/4/2013	11/6/2013	2	27	1
1980	1683	F	5	60	140	chronic obstructive pulmonary disease	MEDICAL	4	11/22/2013	11/24/2013	2	16	1
1981	1683	F	5	61	420	diabetes	MEDICAL	5	12/8/2013	12/9/2013	1	14	1

CHAPTER 7

Exploratory Data Analysis

MARTHA L. SYLVIA

SHANNON MURPHY

Exploratory data analysis (EDA) is both a method for the investigation of data, as well as a set of recommended tools and techniques with the fundamental tenet that the data need to be explored and understood in their most basic form to the point of being meaningful (Smith & Prentice, 1993). EDA encompasses examination of each variable individually and in meaningful combinations, as well as an understanding of the population and/or events of interest. The doctor of nursing practice (DNP) carries out this EDA process prior to the analysis of outcomes measures. The data analysis plan outlines a strategy for collecting data and for measuring outcomes; however, in the EDA phase the goal is to analyze the data without expectations or assumptions about the results. Thus, unexpected findings can be revealed. The exploratory analysis creates meaning from the collected data and provides the structure and preparatory information needed to refine and execute the data analysis plan.

LEARNING OBJECTIVES

After reading this chapter, the DNP should be able to:

- Use exploratory data analysis techniques for variables at any level of measurement
- Describe the distribution of independent, dependent, and descriptive variables
- Identify and define outliers
- Detail methods for managing outliers and nonnormal distributions

EXPLORING DISTRIBUTIONS OF VALUES FOR EACH VARIABLE

During the EDA phase, population and/or event descriptive variables as well as outcome variables are examined. It is important to use tools that allow a display and visualization of all data points when exploring the values for each variable. The following sections describe and illustrate the ideal tables and graphs for displaying each type of data for individual variables, specifically: nominal, dichotomous, ordinal, and continuous formats. In addition to displaying and visualizing the distributions of values for each variable, it is essential to write a concise summary of the interpretation of this study of each variable. This can be done as part of the commenting in syntax, or it can be kept in a separate log. It is crucial to do this during the EDA process because it serves as a progressive documentation of decision making and it aids in writing and presenting the final results of the project.

Nominal Variables

Nominal variables assign a mutually exclusive category (value) to an individual unit of analysis (person in a population or event). Occasionally, the categories of nominal variables are not mutually exclusive and a person/event can be counted in more than one classification. For instance, when grouping age into categories, a person only falls into one category. However, sometimes a variable is set up so that a unit of analysis can have more than one value, as is the case when a question asks the respondent to "choose all of the options that apply." It is best to change that variable to individual yes/no indicators for each of the possible values, if a person can be associated with more than one value for a nominal variable. For example, if one question on a survey asks the respondent to choose each known chronic condition from a list of 10 chronic conditions, it is better to format those data for analysis as a variable for each condition that has a value of yes/no for each individual and explore those data as dichotomous data. Meaningful combinations can also be formed if desired. To illustrate, in the above example it may be informative to create a variable that counts the number of chronic conditions for each individual.

The easiest way to examine categorical data is to look at the frequency of each unit of analysis falling within each classification of the variable. This is done in SPSS by choosing **Analyze → Descriptive Statistics → Frequencies** from the menu bar. The examples that follow use Medicare Claims Synthetic Public Use Files (SynPUFs) for 2010 (Centers for Medicare and Medicaid Services, 2013). These files contain synthetically created claims data file samples for Medicare beneficiaries in each year. Table 7.1 shows the distribution of race.

It is also helpful to look at the data graphically. Two types of charts commonly used to visualize categorical data are bar charts and pie charts. The **Graphs** menu item has all the options for charting. The **Legacy Dialogs** option works like

TABLE 7.1   Percentage of Medicare Patients Within Each Race Category

	Frequency	Percent	Valid Percent	Cumulative Percent
Valid				
White	93433	82.8	82.8	82.8
Black	11947	10.6	10.6	93.4
Others	4841	4.3	4.3	97.7
Hispanic	2590	2.3	2.3	100.0
Total	112811	100.0	100.0	

Output obtained using IBM SPSS (2012).

a Wizard—graphs are created with minimal inputs. The **Chart Builder** allows for more creativity and customization when creating a graph but requires more time in learning the options. Figures 7.1 and 7.2 display the same race information using a bar chart and a pie chart.

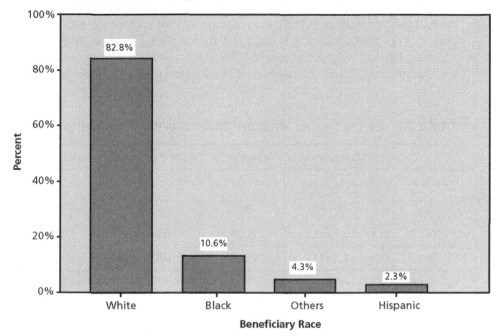

FIGURE 7.1   Percentage of Medicare patients within each race category.
Output obtained using IBM SPSS (2012).

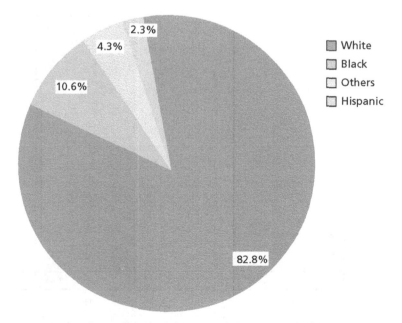

FIGURE 7.2   Percentage of Medicare patients within each race category.
Output obtained using IBM SPSS (2012).

Dichotomous Variables

Investigating individual dichotomous variables, it is easiest to use the frequencies option by choosing **Analyze→Descriptive Statistics→Frequencies** from the menu bar. Under the frequency menu item there is an option to output graphic displays for each of the variables with the percentage results for each of the two categories displayed. This graphic display is not as useful for aiding in providing further understanding beyond what is in the tables. Table 7.2 and Figure 7.3 show an indicator of the chronic condition of Alzheimer's disease in the same Medicare data file.

TABLE 7.2   Percentage of Medicare Patients With Alzheimer's Disease

	Frequency	Percent	Valid Percent	Cumulative Percent
Valid				
Yes	18773	16.6	16.6	16.6
No	94038	83.4	83.4	100.0
Total	112811	100.0	100.0	

Output obtained using IBM SPSS (2012).

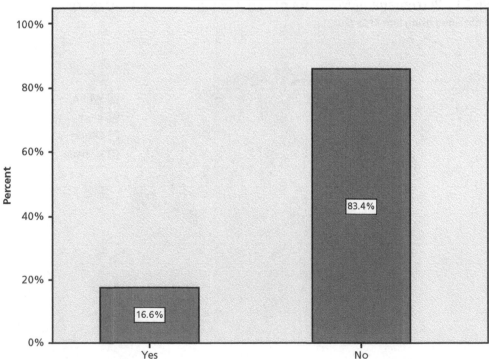

FIGURE 7.3   Percentage of Medicare patients with Alzheimer's disease.

Output obtained using IBM SPSS (2012).

For data with multiple indicator dichotomous variables (e.g., multiple yes/no variables that indicate disease conditions), it is sometimes useful to view the percentages of respondents with each chronic condition within one bar chart. SPSS does not accomplish this easily but there is a way it can be done. Using the Medicare data as an example, the goal is to create a bar chart displaying a separate bar for each condition representing the percentage of the population having each disorder. In SPSS the indicator variables should be coded as 1=yes and 0=no (this is always good practice with yes/no response variables). Choose **Graphs→Legacy Dialogs→Bar→Simple→Summaries of Separate Variables** and move each variable that represents a bar in the chart to the **Bars Represent** section. Next, select each variable and choose **Change Statistic** and convert the statistic to the **Percentage above the Value of 0.** The chart that is output must be formatted with appropriate labels and so forth. Figure 7.4 shows the results of this operation using the Medicare data.

Ordinal Variables

Ordinal variables are explored using tools similar to those employed in examining nominal and dichotomous variables. Statistically testing ordinal variables, the median is the recommended statistic with nonparametric methods; yet,

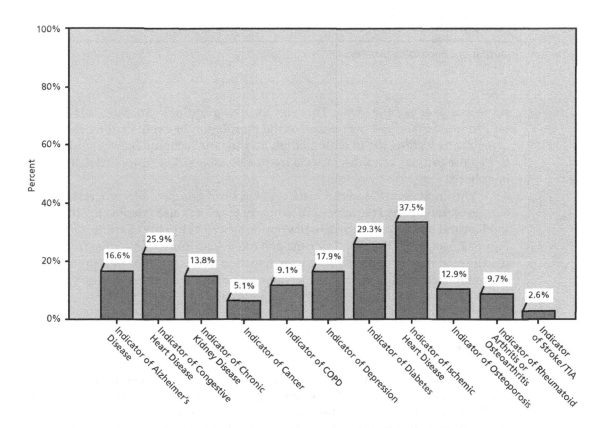

FIGURE 7.4   Percentage of Medicare patients with each chronic condition.

Output obtained using IBM SPSS (2012).

TABLE 7.3   Categorical Age Output Obtained by Running Frequency Command

N				
Valid		112811		
Missing		0		
Mean		3.4217		
Median		3.0000		

	Frequency	Percent	Valid Percent	Cumulative Percent
Valid				
0–49	6718	6.0	6.0	6.0
50–64	10804	9.6	9.6	15.5
65–74	44448	39.4	39.4	54.9
75–84	33295	29.5	29.5	84.4
85–94	14117	12.5	12.5	97.0
95+	3429	3.0	3.0	100.0
Total	112811	100.0	100.0	

Output obtained using IBM SPSS (2012).

some analyses use the mean. Thus, in observing ordinal variables, it is important to understand the percentage of the population or events falling into each category as well as the overall median and mean. Techniques frequently used to explore ordinal variables include frequency tables, descriptive statistics, and bar charts.

Within the same Medicare data, age has been grouped into progressive categories. Running the **Frequency** procedure in SPSS, it is also possible to obtain the median and mean under the **Statistics** option as well as in a bar chart. Table 7.3 and Figure 7.5 show all the output for the age categories from running the frequency distribution that includes the mean, median, and frequency. (For interpretation of the median and mean, the following values represent the age categories: (1) 0–49, (2) 50–64, (3) 65–74, (4) 75–84, (5) 85–94, and (6) 95+.)

Continuous Variables

An investigation of continuous variables includes an assessment of the distribution of values for each variable of interest, as well as outliers in the distribution. Unlike data in categories, continuous variables are best explored using charts and by examining attributes of the variable such as the range, measures of central tendency, and outliers. Histograms, boxplots, and stem-and-leaf plots are all useful ways to display continuous-data elements.

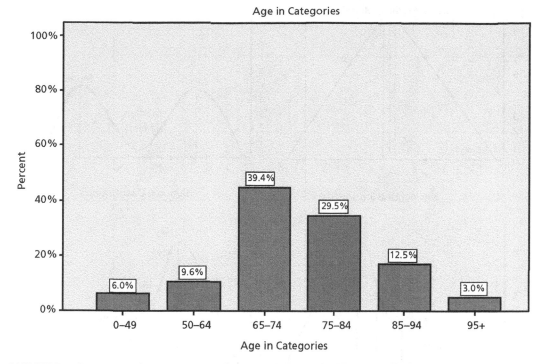

FIGURE 7.5   Categorical age output obtained by running frequency command.

Output obtained using IBM SPSS (2012).

The best way to obtain a variety of information and displays of continuous data in SPSS is to utilize the **Analyze → Descriptive Statistics → Explore** functionality and choose outlier and percentiles for additional **Statistics** and stem and leaf and histogram for additional **Plots**.

ASSESSMENT OF NORMALITY

Parametric statistical tests, which rely on calculations of means and standard deviations of continuous variables, require certain assumptions to be met. One of these assumptions is that the continuous dependent or outcome variable is normally distributed. Assessing normality of a distribution, it is essential to evaluate the distribution of the values along with measures of central tendency (mean, median, and mode).

Continuous data values can be normally distributed, multimodal, skewed negatively or to the left, or skewed positively or to the right. Visualization of the distribution in tandem with the mean, median, and mode usually indicates the distribution that is present. Figure 7.6 displays the four types of distribution. The normal distribution in the top left of the figure is symmetrical and the mean, median, and mode are very close to each other or equal. The bimodal distribution (top right) is one where the mean and median are close to each other or equal but there are two humps in the pattern, causing two modes. A skewed arrangement is one where many values fall to one side of the mean, creating a difference between the median and the mean. The left or negatively skewed distribution (bottom left)

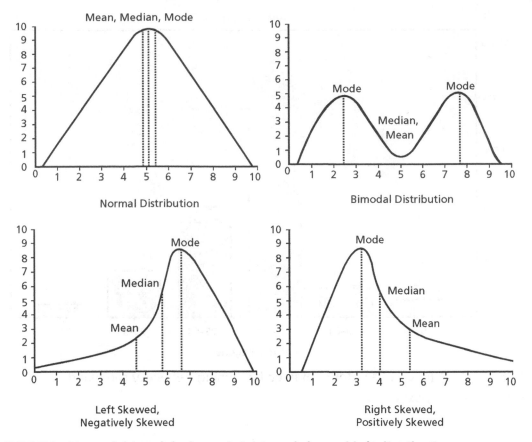

FIGURE 7.6 Normal, bimodal, skewed right, and skewed left distributions.

has a long tail extending to the left, Mean < Median < Mode. The right or positively skewed sequence (bottom right) has a long tail extending to the right, with
the Mean > Median > Mode (Rubin, 2007).

Skewness and kurtosis (kurtosis measures the degree to which a normal
curve is flat or peaked, also expressed as the degree of heaviness of the tails of the
distribution) can be mathematically calculated and assessed to determine the normality of the distribution. SPSS produces a value for kurtosis and skewness by running the **Explore** command. Skewness is a measure of the arrangements of values
in relationship to the mean; in other words, it is a measure of symmetry around the
mean. A skewness statistic close to zero is indicative of a normal curve; the larger
the statistic, the more skewed the distribution. Kurtosis is measured by looking at
the relationship among the mean, standard deviation, and range. A negative value
represents a curve that is flat and widely dispersed (heavy tails), whereas a positive value represents a curve that is highly peaked and narrow (light tails; Rubin,
2007). Measuring the effects of translating evidence into practice, perfectly normal
distributions of outcome variables are not common. These appraisals of normality
are meant to be guidelines and offer a way to describe the divisions of important
continuous descriptive and outcome variables.

The Kolmogorov–Smirnov Test and the Shapiro–Wilk Test are also used to
determine the normality of the distribution of the values of a continuous variable.
The results indicate whether the observed distribution is significantly different from

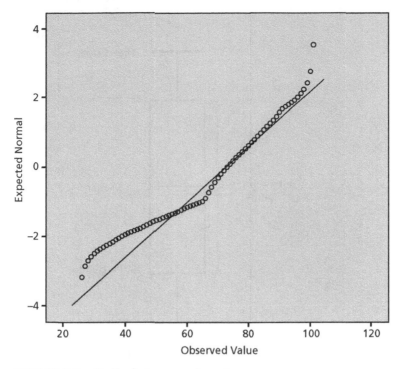

FIGURE 7.7   Q-Q plot example using age.
Output obtained using IBM SPSS (2012).

a standard normal distribution. When the p value for the statistic is less than .05, it means that the observed distribution is significantly different from a normal distribution. It is crucial to note that with large sample sizes the Kolmogorov–Smirnov Test is likely to be significant, with small variations to the perfectly shaped normal curve (Pallant, 2013). Judgment about whether to use parametric statistics in the case of large sample sizes should take all factors into consideration. The results of the Kolmogorov–Smirnov Test are output in the **Explore** function described earlier.

The **Explore** command also produces a Q-Q (Q is quantile) plot for assessment of normality. The Q-Q plot produces a diagonal line that, if the distribution of the data points are normal, the observed data would follow. The more deviant the observed data are from the diagonal Q-Q plot line, the farther away from a normal distribution are the values for the variable (Pallant, 2013). Figure 7.7 shows an example of the Q-Q plot for age in years in the Medicare SynPuf data set. In this example the plot points are closely in line with the diagonal line suggesting a normal distribution.

ASSESSMENT OF OUTLIERS

An outlier is an extreme value in a distribution. At this point the data cleaning process is complete and, therefore, outliers should not be the result of messy data. In some exploratory analyses outliers are determined based on the distance of the value from the mean. A normal distribution by definition contains values under the curve that are within as much as three standard deviations from the mean. Based on the normal distribution, some studies consider values that are greater than two to three standard deviations from the mean to be outliers.

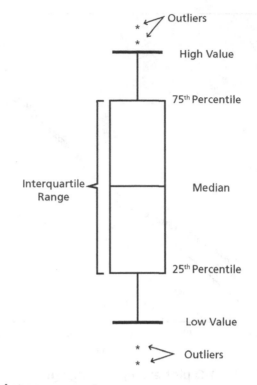

FIGURE 7.8   Boxplot components.
Adapted from Few (2009).

A better way to determine whether a value is an outlier is to base that decision on the distribution itself versus the mean of the distribution; this conclusion relies more heavily on the median as the center of the sequence. By these guidelines a value is considered an outlier if it is positioned greater than 1.5 times the value of the 75th percentile in a distribution (Smith & Prentice, 1993). The box-plot displays outlier values as those that lie above or below each "whisker" (the high and low value in Figure 7.8). The decision of whether to classify a data point as an outlier within a distribution requires judgment on the part of the DNP. Considering measures of central tendency, the mean rather than the median is much more sensitive to outliers; hence, it is important to assess both the mean and median individually and in relationship to each other.

USING GRAPHS TO EXPLORE CONTINUOUS VARIABLES

Histograms, boxplots, and stem-and-leaf plots are three types of graphic displays of data values that are beneficial for exploring continuous variables. The x axis of the histogram contains discrete intervals or bins of values. These intervals: do not overlap, are preferred to be of equal size, and touch each other to indicate the continuous nature of the data. The y axis indicates the frequency or percentage of the values in each bin (Few, 2009). The histogram in Figure 7.9 shows that the distribution of those who are over the age of 65 is somewhat normally distributed, with a slight skew to the right and some patients reaching the age of 100 or more. The mean age is 74.6 with a standard deviation of 6.1.

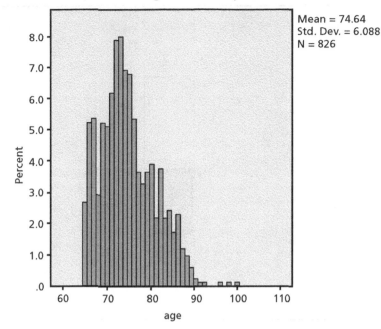

FIGURE 7.9 Histogram example.

Output obtained using IBM SPSS (2012).

Boxplots, also called box and whisker plots, are used, in addition, to show the distribution of values for a variable. The y axis on the boxplot represents values of the continuous variable and the boxplot itself is the distribution of those values. Figure 7.8 illustrates the format of the boxplot along with each component. The boxplot provides a great deal of useful information, including:

- The midspread or the range of the middle 50% of values (interquartile range)
- The median
- The 25th percentile, or the points on or above where 75% of the values reside and on or below where 25% of the values reside
- The 75th percentile, or the points on or above where 25% of the values reside and on or below where 75% of the values reside
- The highest value within 1.5 times the highest point of the interquartile range (high value in Figure 7.8, also called the whisker of the boxplot)
- The lowest value within 1.5 times the lowest point of the interquartile range (low value in Figure 7.8, also called the whisker of the boxplot)
- The outliers (Few, 2009)

Figure 7.10 shows the same data as in Figure 7.9 but displayed in a boxplot instead of a histogram. The boxplot adds to the information in the histogram by showing the median to be at 74, with an interquartile range of 69.5 to 78.4 and three outlier values greater than 95.

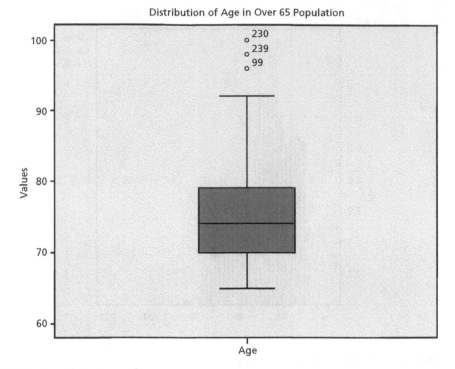

FIGURE 7.10   Boxplot example.

Output obtained using IBM SPSS (2012).

Stem-and-leaf plots are an ideal way to display detailed numerical data within a summarized graphical format. The view and resulting distribution are most similar to a histogram. Each individual value for a variable is translated as a combination of the stem and leaf, with the digits to the left of the line representing the stem and the digits to the right of the line representing the leaf (Few, 2009). Figure 7.11 displays the same age data from Figures 7.9 and 7.10 but in a stem-and-leaf plot. In this plot the frequency of values for each line is displayed. The "Stem width: 10" result means that each stem value is multiplied by 10 (e.g., the 6 represents 60). Each leaf is added to the stem to get the value (e.g., in the first row, each 5 for the leaf along with the 6 for the stem represents the value of 65). The output also indicates that each leaf is equal to 2 cases. When the frequency of values is odd, the highest even number of values closest to the frequency is used to indicate the number of values. For example, there are 87 values of "66" and "67" and there are 43 leaves in that row, when doubled (because each leaf represents 2 cases), that equal 86. When the frequency of values is less than 4, the "&" is used to indicate 1 case being represented.

The stem- and leaf-digit widths vary depending on the distribution of the values for the chosen variable. Regardless of the size of the values, guidelines for the stem and leaves are to assign from one to two digits to the stem and from one to three digits to the leaf (Few, 2009). However, not all software (including SPSS) allows the flexibility to apply these guidelines.

Age Stem-and-Leaf Plot

Frequency	Stem		Leaf
22	6	.	5555555555
87	6	.	66666666666666666666667777777777777777777777
67	6	.	888888888888899999999999999999999
93	7	.	000000000000000000001111111111111111111111111
131	7	.	222222222222222222222222222222222333333333333333333333333333333333
113	7	.	444444444444444444444444444444455555555555555555555555555555
74	7	.	66666666666666666666667777777777777777
57	7	.	88888888888889999999999999999
50	8	.	00000000000000000111111111
49	8	.	2222222222222223333333333
34	8	.	444444444445555555
29	8	.	66666666677777
13	8	.	888899
3	9	.	0&
1	9	.	&
3 Extremes	(>=96)		

Stem width: 10
Each leaf: 2 case(s)
& denotes fractional leaves.

FIGURE 7.11   Stem-and-leaf plot example.

Output obtained using IBM SPSS (2012).

PUTTING IT ALL TOGETHER: EXPLORING CONTINUOUS VARIABLES

The output from the **Explore** command provides a great deal of information about the distribution of a continuous variable. Tables 7.4, 7.5, and 7.6 and Figure 7.12 show the output from analyzing the variable "Age in Years" within the Medicare data set.

Figure 7.12 and Table 7.4 indicate that the mean (72.7) and the median (73.0) for age are very similar. The value for skewness is -0.82, demonstrating that the curve is slightly skewed. The value for kurtosis is 1.48, showing a more peaked and narrow curve. The Kolmogorov–Smirnov statistic indicates that the data are significantly different from that of a normal distribution ($p < .001$). This is a very large sample size, so these results are sensitive to very small deviations from a normal distribution.

The highest value for age in the distribution is 101 and the lowest value for age is 26, with a range of 75. The standard deviation is 12.59. The 5% trimmed mean is a calculation of the mean with the top and bottom 5% of the values for age not included. This value represents a difference in means of 0.61 (73.34–72.73), indicating that extreme outliers are not having a strong impact on the mean. Graphic displays are also helpful in understanding the distribution of age.

The graphical displays for "Age in Years" provide validation of the descriptive table information but also give more detailed information about the distribution. The sequence is left or negatively skewed, with a remarkable jump in the frequency of Medicare recipients over the age of 65. The Medicare program is most available to U.S. citizens over the age of 65, so this pattern is representative of the entire Medicare population. If age were cut off at the eligibility age for retired seniors, the distribution would look different—the majority of enrollees would be between 65 and 80 years old, with a division that is right or positively skewed.

Presenting the final results of EDA, it is vital to choose the appropriate type of graph along with the most pertinent descriptive information. These are matters of preference on the part of the DNP; nonetheless, they are also determined based on the display that best and most efficiently communicates meaningful findings. These points are discussed in greater detail in Chapter 9.

TABLE 7.4   Descriptive Output for Age in Years: Statistics

		Statistic	Standard Error
Age in years	Mean	72.73	.037
	95% confidence interval for mean		
	Lower bound	72.66	
	Upper bound	72.80	
	5% trimmed mean	73.34	
	Median	73.00	
	Variance	158.472	
	Std. deviation	12.589	
	Minimum	26	
	Maximum	101	
	Range	75	
	Interquartile range	14	
	Skewness	–.820	.007
	Kurtosis	1.483	.015

Output obtained using IBM SPSS (2012).

TABLE 7.5   Descriptive Output for Age in Years: Extreme Values

		Case Number	Value
Age in years	Highest		
	1	2608	101
	2	2666	101
	3	9260	101
	4	9578	101
	5	9915	101[a]
	Lowest		
	1	111417	26
	2	111011	26
	3	110031	26
	4	109707	26
	5	109495	26[b]

[a]Only a partial list of cases with the value 101 are shown in the table of upper extremes. [b]Only a partial list of cases with the value 26 are shown in the table of lower extremes.

TABLE 7.6   Descriptive Output for Age in Years: Tests of Normality

	Kolmogorov-Smirnov[a]		
	Statistic	df	Significance
Age in years	.134	112811	.000

[a]Lilliefors significance correction.

Output obtained using IBM SPSS (2012).

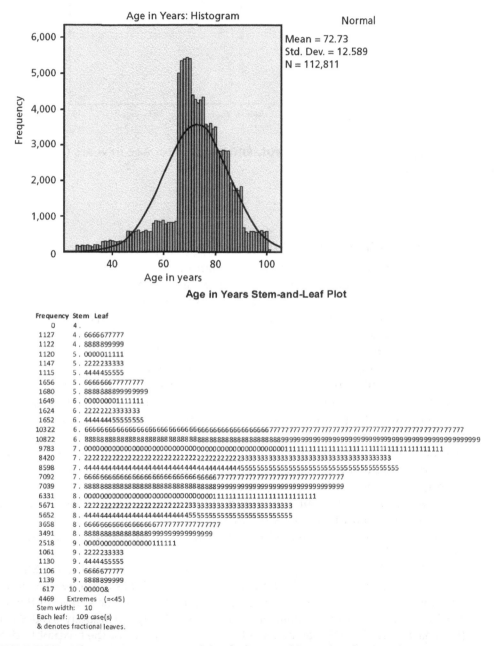

FIGURE 7.12   Histogram, stem-and-leaf plot, and boxplot for age in years.

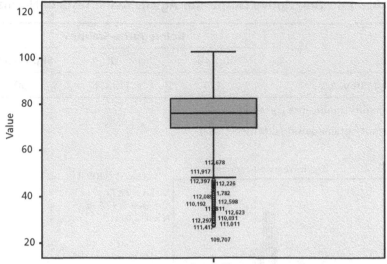

FIGURE 7.12 **Histogram, stem-and-leaf plot, and boxplot for age in years (*continued*).**
Output obtained using IBM SPSS (2012).

THE SPECIAL CASE OF COST AND UTILIZATION DATA

The work of QI through evidence translation often requires that the impact on health care costs and/or utilization be measured as outcomes. It is difficult to perform parametric statistical testing of means for some of these measures because the data often are *not* normally distributed. For instance, examining total costs of health care for patients for a 1-year period—depending on the morbidity of the population—there can be anywhere from 5% to 30% of the population having no health care costs at all during the year. Additionally, when it comes to health care costs and utilization, approximately 20% of patients in a population can account for 80% of the total health care costs for the population (Ehrlich, Kofke-Egger, & Udow-Phillips, 2010). This means that in addition to the problem of many zero costs, the distribution of costs for a population can also have 15% to 25% of values that are greater than three standard deviations (SDs) from the mean of costs for that population. The distribution problem is even greater when reducing the time frame for examining costs from years to months. Utilization variables such as number of hospitalizations and number of emergency room (ER) visits behave similarly. Tables 7.7, 7.8, and 7.9 and Figure 7.13 display this issue in the distribution of costs for Medicare recipients in the SynPUFs.

The total costs of care per year for 19% of this sample of 112,811 Medicare beneficiaries are $0. The distribution of costs is highly right skewed with a mode of $0, a median of $1,180, and a mean (SD) of $3,118 ($6,503). The spread of the middle 50% of the values (interquartile range) is $2,903 (approximately $100–$3,000) (the chart editor in SPSS can be used to expand the y axis of the boxplot to determine this range), and more than 6,000 of the cases have costs larger than two SDs

TABLE 7.7   Key Output From Explore Function for Total Costs per Year for Medicare Beneficiaries: Statistics

		Statistic	Standard Error
Total costs per year	Mean	$3,118.44	$19.362

	95% confidence interval for mean
	    Lower bound
	    Upper bound
		$3,080.49
		$3,156.39	

	5% trimmed mean	$2,049.19	
	Median	$1,180.00	
	Variance	42292172.18	
	Std. deviation	$6,503.243	
	Minimum	$0	
	Maximum	$135,630	
	Range	$135,630	
	Interquartile range	$2,960	
	Skewness	5.535	.007
	Kurtosis	45.545	.015

Output obtained using IBM SPSS (2012).

TABLE 7.8   Key Output From Explore Function for Total Costs per Year for Medicare Beneficiaries: Extreme Values

		Case Number	Value
Total costs per year	Highest		
	1	112753	$135,630
	2	112587	$122,750
	3	112548	$120,030
	4	112355	$113,430
	5	112350	$113,390
	Lowest		
	1	24244	$0
	2	24243	$0
	3	24242	$0
	4	24241	$0
	5	24240	$0[a]

[a]Only a partial list of cases with the value $0 are shown in the table of lower extremes.

TABLE 7.9   Key Output From Explore Function for Total Costs per Year for Medicare Beneficiaries: Tests of Normality

	Kolmogorov-Smirnov[a]		
	Statistic	df	Significance
Total costs per year	.316	112811	.000

[a]Lilliefors significance correction.

from the mean. The mean value of $3,118 is highly influenced by the large amount of values at $0 and the large amount of extreme values at the high end. Therefore, this cost variable does not meet the assumptions for normality necessary for parametric statistical testing.

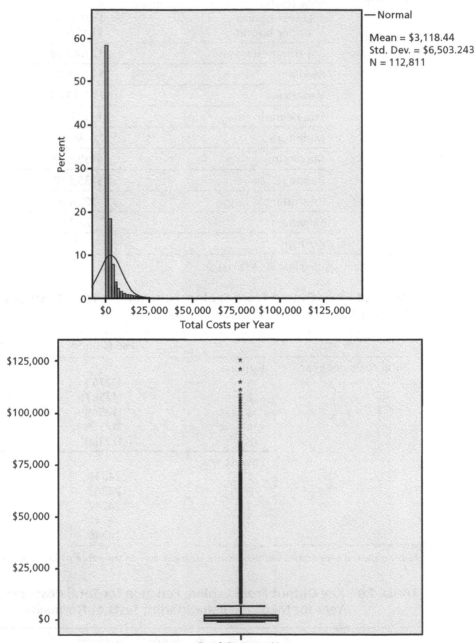

FIGURE 7.13   Key output from Explore function for total costs per year for Medicare beneficiaries.

```
Frequency Stem      Leaf
32012      0 . 00000000000000000000000000000000000000000000000000000000000000000000000000000000000000000000000000001111111111111
5794       0 . 222222222333333333
4999       0 . 4444444455555555
4851       0 . 6666666677777777
4687       0 . 88888889999999
4463       1 . 00000001111111
4081       1 . 2222222333333
3829       1 . 444444555555
3691       1 . 666666777777
3190       1 . 8888899999
3020       2 . 0000011111
2661       2 . 22223333
2491       2 . 44445555
2158       2 . 6666777
2064       2 . 888999
1786       3 . 000111
1526       3 . 2233
1447       3 . 4455
1321       3 . 6677
1167       3 . 8899
1106       4 . 0011
1030       4 . 2233
918        4 . 45
787        4 . 67
710        4 . 89
665        5 . 01
629        5 . 23
607        5 . 45
516        5 . 67
424        5 . 89
469        6 . 01
428        6 . 23
435        6 . 45          11284.00 Extremes (>=7510)
353        6 . 67          Stem width: 1000
356        6 . 88&         Each leaf: 321 case(s); & denotes fractional leaves.
345        7 . 1&
345        7 . 2&
166        7 . &
```

FIGURE 7.13   Key output from Explore function for total costs per year for Medicare beneficiaries (*continued*).

Output obtained using IBM SPSS (2012).

MANAGING OUTLIERS AND NONNORMAL DISTRIBUTIONS

If the data are normally distributed with a minimal amount of outlier values, it is important to assess the reason for the outlier values. The first question to ask: "Are the outlier value(s) valid data points?" If the outlier(s) are valid data points, one way to handle them is to explore the variable and potentially analyze the results both with and without the outlier(s). When the outlier value(s) are valid data points, these data points provide meaning to the final results that should not be lost.

Figure 7.14 shows a final display of cost data that allows the reporting of the distribution of costs with and without an extreme outlier value. The gray dots represent individual values for the variable cost and the black diamonds represent the mean. In this example, the intervention group of a QI initiative for highly morbid patients with diabetes contained one patient with costs above $100,000 for a 6-month period, due to receiving a kidney transplant. The program was not designed to prevent an imminent transplant; hence, the best way to handle reporting the results is to explain the outlier and report further results without the outlier.

Even removing the extreme outlier value over $100,000 in Figure 7.14, the distribution of costs for both groups and each group individually remains positively (right) skewed. When this is the case and many outlier values are causing a distribution to be skewed, other solutions should be sought for analysis. Essentially, most analyses handle this situation in one or a combination of four possible ways. One way to manage this situation is to use statistical techniques such as transforming the scale of an outcome variable prior to analysis. The second option is to use nonparametric statistical tests that rely on the distribution or ranking of the values as opposed to the mean. A third method is to change the continuous variable into a categorical or dichotomous variable and, similar

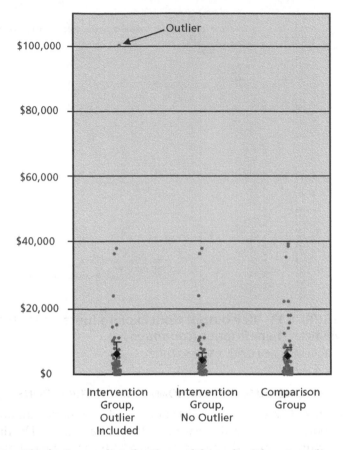

FIGURE 7.14   Displaying a distribution with and without outliers.

to the second option, use a nonparametric statistic such as chi-square to analyze outcomes. The fourth, and least desirable, step is to impute new values for outliers and/or remove their values completely from the analysis. If utilized, this last option must be well justified. In trying to decide which method(s) to use, it is best to consult with a biostatistician.

SUMMARY

EDA is necessary for understanding the distributions and characteristics of descriptive, demographic, and key outcomes before analyzing project results. EDA equips the DNP with a thorough comprehension of each variable and provides sound justification for the statistics chosen and methods employed to measure successful outcomes.

REFERENCES

Centers for Medicare and Medicaid Services. (2013, July 10). CMS.Gov. *Medicare claims synthetic public use files (SynPUFs)*. Retrieved August 13, 2013, from http://www .cms.gov/Research-Statistics-Data-and-Systems/Statistics-Trends-and-Reports/ SynPUFs

Ehrlich, E., Kofke-Egger, H., & Udow-Phillips, M. (2010). *Health care cost drivers: Chronic disease, comorbidity, and health risk factors in the U.S. and Michigan.* Ann Arbor, MI: Center for Healthcare Research & Transformation.

Few, S. (2009). *Now you see it.* Oakland, CA: Analytics Press.

IBM. (2012). *IBM SPSS Statistics for Windows, version 21.0.* Armonk, NY: Author.

Pallant, J. (2013). *SPSS survival manual.* New York, NY: McGraw-Hill.

Rubin, A. (2007). *Statistics for evidence-based practice and evaluation.* Belmont, CA: Brooks/Cole.

Smith, A. F., & Prentice, D. A. (1993). Exploratory data analysis. In G. Kereen & C. Lewis (Eds.), *A handbook for data analysis in the behavioral sciences: Statistical issues* (pp. 349–389). Hillsdale, NJ: Lawrence Erlbaum.

CASE STUDY

CASE STUDY EXAMPLE: EXPLORATORY DATA ANALYSIS (EDA)

DESCRIPTIVE VARIABLES FOR OLDER COMMUNITY-DWELLING PATIENTS WITH DIABETES

- Overall N = 392
    - Intervention group—208 patients
    - Comparison group—184 patients
- Age
    - Age has a slightly positively skewed distribution. The overall population mean is 74.7, the median is 74.0, and the mode is 73.0. The minimum age is 65 and the maximum age is 100. The skewness statistic is .672 and the kurtosis statistic is .310. The visualization of the distribution, the positions of the mean, median, and mode—as well as the skewness and kurtosis statistics—all indicate a curve that is normal; however, the significant Kolmogorov–Smirnov statistic indicates a nonnormal curve. The breakdown by group is similar to the distribution overall. Further statistical testing is necessary to confirm this similarity.

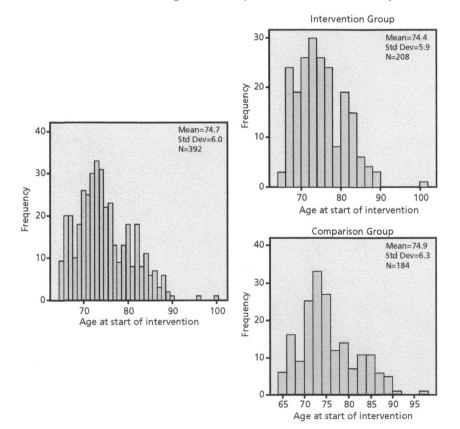

- Gender
    - In the overall population, 58.7% are men and 41.3% are women. In the intervention group, 61.1% are men and 38.9% are women; in the comparison group, 56.0% are men and 44.0% are women.

- Race
  - For all patients, 44.6% are Black, 52.3% are White, and a small percentage (3.1%) are Hispanic.

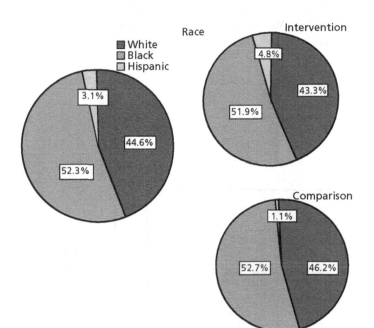

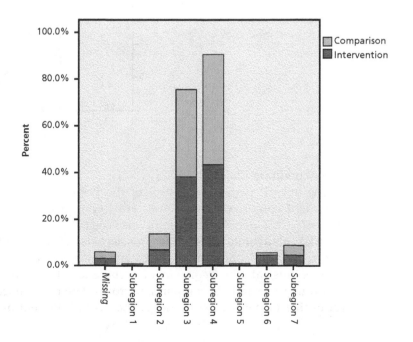

- Morbidity level
  - Taking into account all patients, 97.7% are in the "moderate risk" to "very high risk" morbidity levels, with the highest percentage (69.6%) in the "high risk" or "very high risk" categories. Considered as a continuous variable, the mean, median, and mode of the distribution of scores is 4.0 (on a scale of 0–5). None of the patients had a value of 0 (no risk) or 1 (very low risk). The intervention group has a higher percentage of patients in the "high risk" and "very high risk" morbidity categories than the comparison group (74% vs. 64.7%).

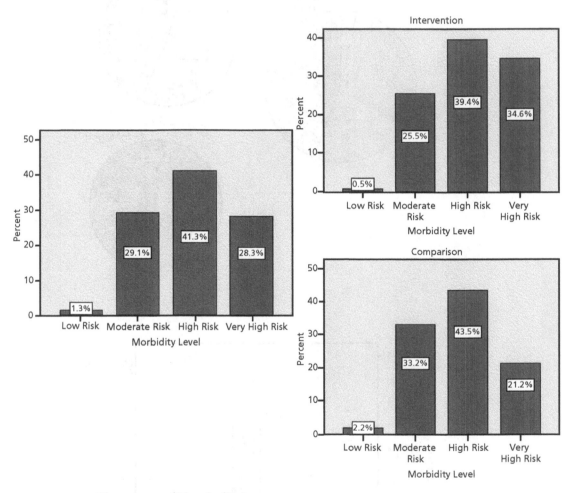

- Chronic condition indicators
  - In the overall population, 100% of the patients have diabetes. The most prevalent comorbidities, overall, are hypertension (82.1%), lipid disorders (75.0%), degenerative joint disease (34.7%), ischemic heart disease (26.8%), glaucoma (26.8%), atherosclerosis (25.8%), and obesity (18.6%). The remaining condition prevalence is below 15% for each disorder. The graphs illustrate the frequency of occurrence of comorbidities in the intervention group and the comparison group. The prevalence of comorbidities for each group is similar to that of the overall population.

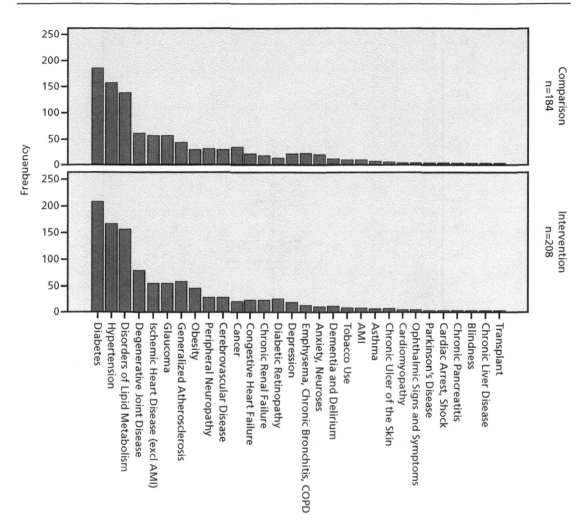

OUTCOME VARIABLES FOR OLDER COMMUNITY-DWELLING PATIENTS WITH DIABETES

- Hemoglobin A1C (HbA1C) value 6 months following the start of the intervention
  - The distribution of HbA1C values in the postperiod is right skewed, with the Mean > Median > Mode. The skewness value of 2.4 and the kurtosis value of 9.0 also indicate a skewed, peaked pattern. There are many values beyond the 75th percentile and also beyond the whiskers of the boxplot. Nevertheless, these values represent valid HbA1C patient measurements and must be considered in measuring the success of this outcome measure. Alternatives to parametric statistical testing of means need to be contemplated when testing this outcome measure.

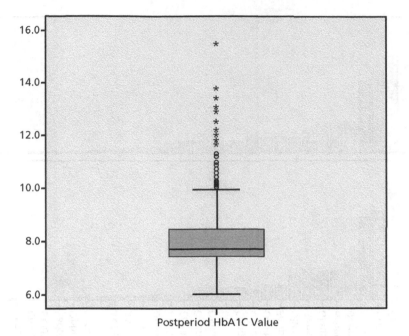

Postperiod HbA1C Value

Mean = 8.1
Median = 7.7
Mode = 7
Std Dev = 1.3
N = 392

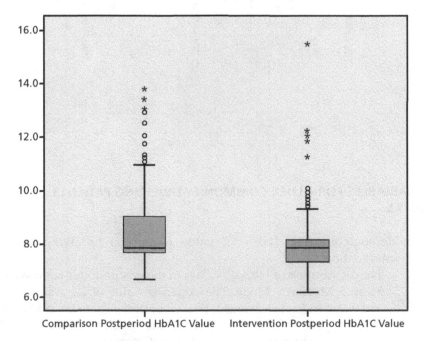

Comparison Postperiod HbA1C Value   Intervention Postperiod HbA1C Value

Mean = 8.3   Mean = 7.9
Median = 7.7   Median = 7.7
Mode = 7   Mode = 7
Std Dev = 1.4   Std Dev = 1.2
N = 184   N = 208

- Pre/post difference in HbA1C value
  - The distribution of the differences in HbA1C values from the preperiod to the postperiod has a normal-shaped, high-peaked distribution with some extreme values at each end. The overall mean difference is 0.3, the median is 0.4, and the mode is 1.2. The skewness value of -0.3 and the kurtosis value of 2.7 indicate a normal curve whose top is slightly more peaked.

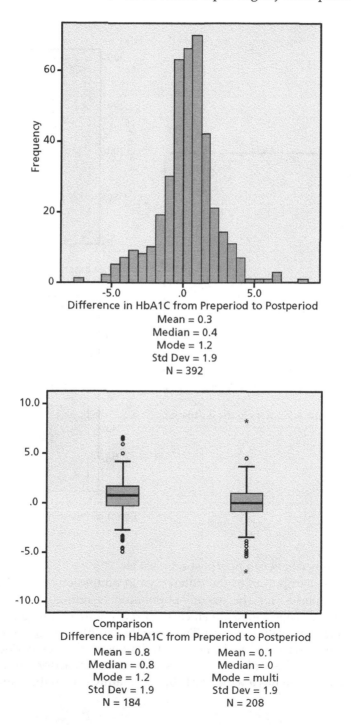

Difference in HbA1C from Preperiod to Postperiod
Mean = 0.3
Median = 0.4
Mode = 1.2
Std Dev = 1.9
N = 392

Difference in HbA1C from Preperiod to Postperiod

Comparison	Intervention
Mean = 0.8	Mean = 0.1
Median = 0.8	Median = 0
Mode = 1.2	Mode = multi
Std Dev = 1.9	Std Dev = 1.9
N = 184	N = 208

- Number of admissions in the postperiod
  - The distribution of admissions in the postperiod is highly right skewed, with many patients having no admissions (mean = 0.4, median and mode = 0). This distribution is similar for the intervention and the comparison groups. Alternatives to parametric statistical testing of means need to be considered when testing this outcome measure.

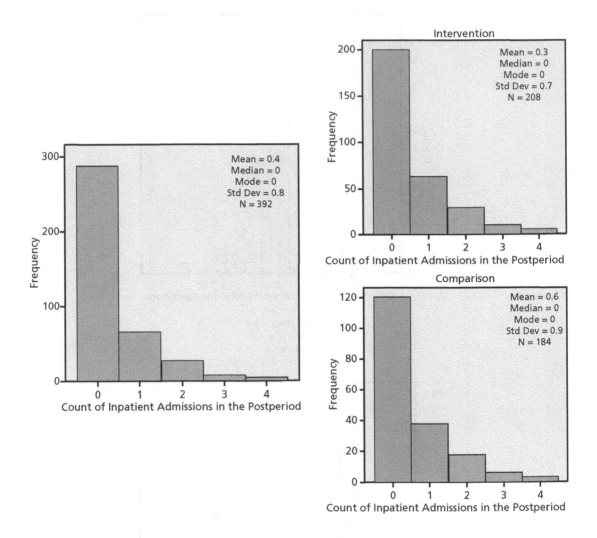

- Difference between pre/post-admissions
  - The distribution of the differences in admissions from the preperiod to the postperiod for the overall population is normally distributed (the mean, median, and mode are all close to zero) with a high, narrow peak representing many values at zero. There are three outliers in the distribution that have four, seven, and eight fewer admissions in the postperiod compared to the preperiod. All of these outliers are in the comparison group. The comparison group also has a wider distribution mainly due to the outlier values.

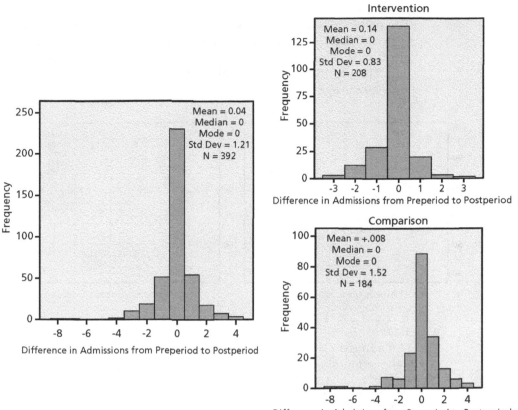

- Indicator of an admission in the postperiod
  - In the overall population, 26.8% have an admission in the postperiod. In the intervention group, 19.7% have an admission in the postperiod. In the comparison group, 34.8% have an admission in the postperiod.

DESCRIPTIVE AND OUTCOME VARIABLES FOR INPATIENT ADMISSIONS (DIABETES READMISSIONS PREVENTION INITIATIVE)

There are a total of 4,108 admissions in the data set for the community-dwelling patients with diabetes who are enrolled in Care1 health plan for 1 full year following the implementation of the readmissions prevention initiative. Of these total 4,108 admissions, 722 are readmissions. Descriptive variables are explored for the total of the 4,108 admissions and the 722 readmissions.

- Patients
  - A total of 2,470 patients account for the 4,108 total admissions.
  - Of the total 2,470 patients, 13% ($n = 309$) account for the 722 readmissions. This leaves 87% of the total patients with no readmission.

- Age
  - The pattern of age is right skewed for all admissions and for readmissions, with the Mode < Median < Mean. The skewness and kurtosis statistic values of 2.0 and 7.0 respectively confirm that this is a skewed and peaked distribution. This is due to the high number of values at 50 years of age and the outliers over the age of 70.

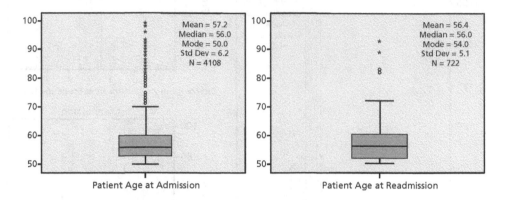

Patient Age at Admission   Patient Age at Readmission

- Gender
  - (All admissions by women—55.3%)
  - (All readmissions by women—43.4%) (No graphic shown.)

- DRGs (diagnostic-related groups)
  - A wide variety of DRGs account for admissions and readmissions, with the highest-frequency DRG (chronic obstructive pulmonary disease [COPD]) associated with only 6.4% of overall admissions. Only the top 15 frequent DRGs are shown in the following table. A total of 237 DRGs are present in all the admissions and a total of 156 DRGs are present in the readmissions. It is difficult to glean pertinent information about the readmissions from the DRG descriptions.

Total Admissions N = 4108			Readmissions N = 722		
DRG	Frequency	Percent	DRG	Frequency	Percent
Chronic obstructive pulmonary disease	264	6.4	Chronic obstructive pulmonary disease	53	7.3
Heart failure	156	3.8	Heart failure	41	5.7
Knee joint replacement	137	3.3	Pulmonary edema & respiratory failure	25	3.5
Septicemia & disseminated infections	104	2.5	Septicemia & disseminated infections	25	3.5
Other pneumonia	102	2.5	Disorders of pancreas except malignancy	19	2.6
Cellulitis & other bacterial skin infections	98	2.4	Electrolyte disorders except hypovolemia related	17	2.4

(continued)

Total Admissions N = 4108			Readmissions N = 722		
DRG	Frequency	Percent	DRG	Frequency	Percent
Disorders of pancreas except malignancy	83	2.0	Renal failure	17	2.4
Renal failure	81	2.0	Cellulitis & other bacterial skin infections	15	2.1
Hip joint replacement	77	1.9	Other pneumonia	15	2.1
Pulmonary edema & respiratory failure	67	1.6	Diabetes	14	1.9
Cerebrovascular accident (CVA) & precerebral occlusion w/ infarct	66	1.6	Peptic ulcer & gastritis	14	1.9
Cardiac arrhythmia & conduction disorders	63	1.5	Hepatic coma & other major acute liver disorders	13	1.8
Diabetes	62	1.5	HIV w major HIV related conditions	13	1.8
Electrolyte disorders except hypovolemia related	56	1.4	HIV w multiple major HIV related conditions	13	1.8
Seizure	56	1.4	Peripheral & other vascular disorders	13	1.8

- Bed type
  - The majority of admissions and readmissions occur within two bed types (medical and intensive care). It is unlikely that there is enough granularity in this variable to gather any important revealing information about readmissions.

Bed Type	All Admissions (%)	Readmissions (%)
Medical	81.5	79.5
Intensive care unit	16.1	18.0
Acute rehab	1.2	1.5
Psychiatric	0.7	0.6
Other	0.3	0.4
Obstetrics	0.2	0.0
Subacute	0.1	0.0

- Readmissions
  - Of the overall 4,108 admissions, 722 are readmissions. This is a rate of 17.6%.

CHAPTER 8

Outcomes Data Analysis

MARTHA L. SYLVIA

SHANNON MURPHY

Outcomes data analysis (ODA) is the final step in data management. Of all of the phases of data management, it is perhaps the easiest after all the work that has gone into preparing and analyzing the data to this point. If the translational project does not use groups for comparison, the analysis of outcomes is solely descriptive or may use a comparison to some type of benchmark or predetermined goal. When the Doctor of Nursing Practice (DNP) uses some type of comparison group in the translational project, statistical testing is done to determine the success of outcomes compared to another group or the same group at a different point in time. This is all predetermined in the data analysis plan.

LEARNING OBJECTIVES

After reading this chapter, the DNP should be able to:

- Use SPSS to perform bivariate statistical tests
- Employ techniques for quantifying uncertainty in statistical estimates
- Identify confounding variables
- Describe the unit of analysis and any subgroups
- Perform bivariate statistical testing of outcomes measures
- Utilize multivariate methods to adjust for confounding
- Determine the success of interventions based on the outcomes

BIVARIATE STATISTICAL TESTING

Bivariate statistical testing is defined as the study of the relationship between two variables. In Chapter 7 univariate (one variable) distributions are explored. The data analysis plan developed in Chapter 4 describes the bivariate statistical test that would be used to statistically evaluate outcomes between two groups. Common bivariate tests that are utilized to investigate differences between independent groups are the independent *t*-test, analysis of variance (ANOVA), and chi-square. The bivariate paired *t*-test is most commonly employed to test paired data in the same individuals. Correlation is also used to study the relationship between two variables.

There are assumptions required for the use of certain bivariate statistical tests that are described briefly in Chapter 2. Utilization of the independent *t*-test, paired *t*-test, and ANOVA depends on the normal distribution of the variable for which the mean is being calculated (dependent or outcome variable). Chi-square is a nonparametric test and does not depend on assumptions of normality but does depend on having a minimum amount of observations in each combination of values for the variables of interest. Assumptions for correlation are that the appropriate level of measurement for each variable is used for the chosen correlation test.

Independent *T*-Test

In SPSS all the statistical functions are found under the **Analyze** menu item. To run the independent *t*-test, select **Analyze → Compare Means → Independent Samples *T*-Test**. Choose the appropriate variable that indicates groups under the 'grouping variable' (assign the data value for each group). Next, pick the appropriate dependent variable under the 'test variable' and run the test. Figure 8.1 shows the output from the *t*-test using the 2010 Medicare Claims Synthetic Public Use Files (SynPUFs) data with pertinent annotated interpretations (Centers for

Group Statistics

	Gender	N	Mean	Std. Deviation	Std. Error Mean
Age in years	Male	50243	71.19	12.601	.056
	Female	62568	73.97	12.441	.050

Mean (SD) age for females is 71.2 (12.6) and for males is 74.0 (12.4).

Independent Samples Test

		Levene's Test for Equality of Variances		*t*-test for Equality of Means						
		F	Sig.	*t*	df	Sig. (2-tailed)	Mean Difference	Std. Error Difference	95% Confidence Interval of the Difference	
Age in years	Equal variances assumed	5.963	.015	−37.096	112809	.000	−2.781	.075	−2.927	−2.634
	Equal variances not assumed			−37.044	107026.177	.000	−2.781	.075	−2.928	−2.633

Levene's test *p*-value is less than .05, indicating a significant difference in the variance of the two groups. If continuing to use the independent *t*-test, the results under "Equal variances not assumed" must be used. However, since the *t*-test assumes equal variances, a nonparametric test should be considered.

This *t*-test *p*-value is less than .05, indicating a significant difference in age between males and females.

FIGURE 8.1 **Annotated output from the independent *t*-test.**
SD, standard deviation.
Source: Pallant (2013).
Output obtained using IBM SPSS (2012).

Medicare and Medicaid Services, 2013). The *t*-test in this example is answering the question of whether mean age is significantly different for women versus men. The 'grouping variable' is gender and the testing variable is age.

ANOVA

To run ANOVA, select **Analyze → Compare Means → One-Way ANOVA**. Pick the appropriate variable that indicates the factor (this is the 'grouping variable') and choose the dependent variable for which the mean is to be tested for each group within the factor. Although the *t*-test is limited to comparisons between two groups, ANOVA can test for differences in means among two or more groups. Figure 8.2 shows the output from the ANOVA using the Medicare SynPUFs data with pertinent

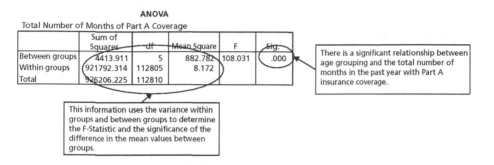

ANOVA

Total Number of Months of Part A Coverage

	Sum of Squares	df	Mean Square	F	Sig.
Between groups	4413.911	5	882.782	108.031	.000
Within groups	921792.314	112805	8.172		
Total	926206.225	112810			

There is a significant relationship between age grouping and the total number of months in the past year with Part A insurance coverage.

This information uses the variance within groups and between groups to determine the F-Statistic and the significance of the difference in the mean values between groups.

Multiple Comparisons

Dependent Variable: Total Number of Months of Part A Coverage
LSD

(I) Age in Categories	(J) Age in Categories	Mean Difference (I-J)	Std. Error	Sig.	95% Confidence Interval Lower Bound	95% Confidence Interval Upper Bound
0-49	50-64	-.054	.044	.222	-.14	.03
	65-74	-.085*	.037	.023	-.16	-.01
	75-84	-.472*	.038	.000	-.55	-.40
	85-94	-.479*	.042	.000	-.56	-.40
	95+	-.243*	.060	.000	-.36	-.13
50-64	0-49	.054	.044	.222	-.03	.14
	65-74	-.031	.031	.311	-.09	.03
	75-84	-.418*	.032	.000	-.48	-.36
	85-94	-.424*	.037	.000	-.50	-.35
	95+	-.189*	.056	.001	-.30	-.08
65-74	0-49	.085*	.037	.023	-.01	.16
	50-64	.031	.031	.311	-.03	.09
	75-84	-.387*	.021	.000	-.43	-.35
	85-94	-.393*	.028	.000	-.45	-.34
	95+	-.158*	.051	.002	-.26	-.06
75-84	0-49	-.472*	.038	.000	.40	.55
	50-64	-.418*	.032	.000	.36	.48
	65-74	.387*	.021	.000	.35	.43
	85-94	-.007	.029	.816	-.06	.05
	95+	.228*	.051	.000	.13	.33
85-94	0-49	.479*	.042	.000	.40	.56
	50-64	.424*	.037	.000	.35	.50
	65-74	.393*	.028	.000	.34	.45
	75-84	.007	.029	.816	-.05	.06
	95+	.235*	.054	.000	.13	.34
95+	0-49	.243*	.060	.000	.13	.34
	50-64	.189*	.056	.001	.08	.30
	65-74	.158*	.051	.002	.06	.26
	75-84	-.228*	.051	.000	-.33	-.13
	85-94	-.235*	.054	.000	-.34	-.13

A significance level of less than 0.05 indicates a significant relationship between the categories of each variable. For instance, here it shows that the mean months of Part A coverage for those in age group 65–74 is significantly different than the mean months of Part A coverage in all other age groups except for the 50–64 category, where the significance level is 0.311.

*The mean difference is significant at the 0.05 level.

FIGURE 8.2   Annotated output from the ANOVA test.
Source: Pallant (2013).
Output obtained using IBM SPSS (2012).

annotated interpretations. The ANOVA in this example is answering the question of whether the mean months of Part A insurance coverage during the previous year differs by age group. The factor variable is 'age grouping' and the dependent variable is 'months of Part A coverage.' Using ANOVA, it is helpful to choose the least significant difference (LSD) post hoc tests in order to determine where the significant relationships lie among values of each variable if they do exist.

Chi-Square

To run chi-square, select **Analyze → Descriptive Statistics → Crosstabs**. It is good practice to put the independent variable in the row section and the dependent variable in the column section. Choose the desired statistic (chi-square) under the statistics option and pick other desired options under the other optional categories. Figure 8.3 shows the output from chi-square using the Medicare SynPUFs data with pertinent annotated interpretations. The chi-square in this example is answering the question of whether the proportion of those with congestive heart failure is significantly different for women versus men. The two variables are 'gender' and 'indicator of congestive heart failure.' Note, when there are more than two values for the independent variable, the chi-square test only indicates that there is a significant difference somewhere; however, further testing is needed to determine specifically the location of that difference.

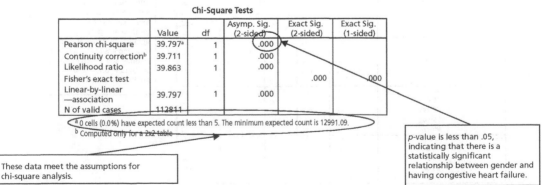

FIGURE 8.3   Annotated output from the chi-square test.

Source: Pallant (2013).

Output obtained using IBM SPSS (2012).

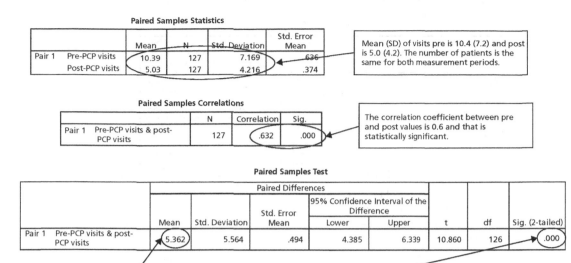

Paired Samples Statistics

		Mean	N	Std. Deviation	Std. Error Mean
Pair 1	Pre-PCP visits	10.39	127	7.169	.636
	Post-PCP visits	5.03	127	4.216	.374

Mean (SD) of visits pre is 10.4 (7.2) and post is 5.0 (4.2). The number of patients is the same for both measurement periods.

Paired Samples Correlations

		N	Correlation	Sig.
Pair 1	Pre-PCP visits & post-PCP visits	127	.632	.000

The correlation coefficient between pre and post values is 0.6 and that is statistically significant.

Paired Samples Test

		Paired Differences							
					95% Confidence Interval of the Difference				
		Mean	Std. Deviation	Std. Error Mean	Lower	Upper	t	df	Sig. (2-tailed)
Pair 1	Pre-PCP visits & post-PCP visits	5.362	5.564	.494	4.385	6.339	10.860	126	.000

There is an average of 5.4 fewer visits in the postperiod compared to the preperiod and that difference is statistically significant.

FIGURE 8.4   Annotated output from the paired *t*-test.
PCP, primary care provider; SD, standard deviation.
Source: Pallant (2013).
Output obtained using IBM SPSS (2012).

Paired *T*-Test

To run the paired *t*-test, select **Analyze → Compare Means → Paired Samples *T*-Test**. Choose the appropriate pair of variables that indicate pre/postmeasurement for the same individuals and place them in the first pair and run the test. Figure 8.4 shows the output from the paired *t*-test using a small test sample of the Medicare SynPUFs patients. The paired *t*-test in this example is answering the question of whether the number of in-person visits to a primary care provider (PCP) changed after an intervention to improve the efficiency of the delivery of primary care services. The paired variables are 'pre-PCP visits' and 'post-PCP visit.'

Correlation

This section reviews the Pearson product-moment correlation (r) procedure used to test the strength and direction of the relationship between two variables that are each measured at the interval or ratio level. Other types of correlation exist for comparison of other levels of measurement. To run the independent *t*-test, select **Analyze → Correlations → Bivariate**. Pick the appropriate variables at the interval or ratio level and enter them into the variables section; choose 'Pearson' under 'Correlation Coefficients.' Figure 8.5 illustrates the results of running a correlation using the Medicare SynPufs data to answer the question of whether there is a relationship between age and total paid amount (note, for the purposes of this example, only costs greater than $500 are used because of the skewed distribution of expenses).

Correlations[a]

		Age in Years	Total Paid by Medicare for Year
Age in years	Pearson correlation	1	.005
	Sig. (2-tailed)		.390
	N	30280	30280
Total paid by Medicare for year	Pearson correlation	.005	1
	Sig. (2-tailed)	.390	
	N	30280	30280

a. Paid total costs > $500 = 1

The significance level of the correlation is > 0.05, meaning that the correlation between "age" and "total paid" is not significant.

The Pearson correlation coefficient value is between -1 and 1 where values of 0 = no correlation and values of +/-1 indicate perfect correlation. This output shows that there is a positive, extremely weak (close to 0 correlation) relationship between "age" and "total paid."

FIGURE 8.5   Annotated output from correlation.
Source: Pallant (2013).
Output obtained using IBM SPSS (2012).

p Values

Chapter 2 defines the *p* value is the same as alpha or the significance level, and it is equal to the percentage chance the conclusion can be drawn that there is a significant statistical difference between groups when in reality there is no significant difference. It is common to use a *p* value of < .05 to determine statistically significant differences between groupings in translational evidence projects. This means that when *p* < .05, there is less than a 5% chance that a statistically significant difference between groups could be reported in error.

DESCRIBING THE UNIT OF ANALYSIS AND DIFFERENCES BETWEEN GROUPS

If the data analysis plan does not have any subgroupings of the unit of analysis (population or events), the unit of analysis is described according to the descriptive variables laid out in the analysis plan. If there are subgroupings that are used for comparison, these subgroups are compared to each other using the chosen descriptive variables to determine if there are any significant differences between groups that may influence outcomes other than the intervention or treatment effect of interest.

Describing the attributes of the unit of analysis, the appropriate statistics should be used. Categorical and dichotomous data are reported as frequencies and percentages. Continuous data are documented using measures of central tendency and, depending on the distribution, are recorded using measures such as the mean, standard deviation, median, minimum, maximum, and/or range. Ordinal data are reported utilizing either frequencies or percentages. They can also be described using measures of central tendency, depending on whether the variable is treated as categorical or continuous.

Comparing subgroupings of the unit of analysis, the appropriate bivariate statistic should be used to determine statistically significant differences between groups on any of the descriptive attributes. It is important to remember that assumptions for using each statistic should be met when doing this comparison. Tables 2.2 and 2.3 in Chapter 2 provide a helpful reference for deciding upon the appropriate statistical test.

Table 8.1 illustrates an example of describing the differences between an intervention group and a comparison group for an evidence-based intervention

TABLE 8.1   Describing the Differences in Subgroupings

Characteristic	Intervention	Comparison	Statistic Used	Statistical Significance
Number in group	970	838	N/A	N/A
Mean age in years (range)	42.92 (18–64)	43.05 (16–64)	Independent t-test	Not significant
% Women	79.79%	72.79%	Chi-square	$p < .05$, significant
% Becoming ineligible	2.78%	8.23%	Chi-square	Not significant
% Low risk	67.53%	67.90%		
% Moderate risk	24.43%	24.82%	Chi-square	Not significant
% High risk	8.04%	7.28%		
% Cardiovascular condition	89.79%	90.21%	Chi-square	Not significant
% Hypertension	78.76%	80.67%	Chi-square	Not significant
% Asthma	42.27%	35.80%	Chi-square	$p < .05$, significant
% Diabetes	39.69%	35.44%	Chi-square	Not significant
% Kidney disease	14.54%	11.93%	Chi-square	Not significant
% COPD	12.89%	16.59%	Chi-square	$p < .05$, significant
% Neurological condition	12.37%	9.07%	Chi-square	$p < .05$, significant
% Peripheral circulatory condition	11.75%	4.18%	Chi-square	$p < .05$, significant
% Kidney failure	2.37%	2.74%	Chi-square	Not significant
% Respiratory failure	1.03%	1.55%	Chi-square	Not significant
% Smoking	45.36%	47.02%	Chi-square	Not significant
% Substance abuse	41.65%	47.61%	Chi-square	$p < .05$, significant

COPD, chronic obstructive pulmonary disease; N/A, not applicable.

to improve outcomes for patients with chronic illness. The first column shows the characteristic that is being measured. The second and third columns exhibit the values for the appropriate summary statistic (percentage or mean) for each characteristic. The fourth column displays the statistic that was used to test the differences in the percentage or mean between the intervention and comparison groups, and the fifth column indicates whether the difference in the summary statistic is statistically significantly different between the two groups.

DESCRIBING UNCERTAINTY

A statistic such as the mean, standard deviation, or proportion is calculated directly from the data collected in the translational project and is, therefore, a "known" number and is referred to as a "point estimate." Uncertainty comes into play when the desire is to understand what the statistic might be for a different sample from the same (or similar) population. Said another way, the point estimate would be different if the same data elements are collected in another sample that meets all the same inclusion and exclusion criteria, in the same setting, with similar characteristics. There are methods to measure this type of uncertainty, attempting to use the sample statistic to estimate what the statistic might be in another sample. It is good practice to include a measure of uncertainty when reporting a point estimate for outcomes.

The most common way to describe uncertainty in a point estimate is to report the confidence interval (CI), usually the 95% CI when the alpha level is .05. A CI is a range of values within which the point estimate would fall (95% of the time, with a 95% CI), if the data are collected in another sample defined by the same inclusion and exclusion criteria, in the same setting, with similar characteristics (Keller & Kelvin, 2013). SPSS provides CIs with mean and proportion point estimates either automatically or by choosing the option when running statistical tests. The best way to obtain the 95% CI for individual means or proportions is to run the **Analyze → Explore** function for the variable of interest.

RECOGNIZING CONFOUNDING

Even the earliest nurse researcher, Florence Nightingale, recognized the effects of confounding on outcome measures and made great strides in measuring and using statistics to adjust for confounding, when examining mortality outcomes among hospitals. In 1861, the mortality rates for hospitals in England were published, with an overall mortality rate of 57% for all hospitals. Separating the mortality rates by the geographic area of the hospital, it was noted that the mortality rates varied between 91% at London hospitals and 39% at county hospitals. Not only did Ms. Nightingale recognize the effect of geographic location on mortality outcomes, but she used this information to make the case for collecting hospital-specific and patient-specific descriptive data to understand more of the factors that may have also had an effect on mortality outcomes. This work contributed to great improvements in hospital conditions and patient outcomes (Nightingale, 1863).

Confounding is the situation where the relationship (or lack of relationship) between the independent variable and the dependent variable is due at least in part to the effects of a third variable, or confounder, that is associated with the independent variable and is a predictor of the dependent variable. Confounding causes a distortion of the true relationship between an independent variable and a dependent variable. In order for a variable to be considered a confounder, it must have an association with the independent variable and with the dependent variable (Fitzmaurice, 2003). The effects of confounding can take either direction in the result of the outcome—confounders can overestimate or underestimate the impact of the intervention on the dependent outcome variable.

In many DNP projects that compare outcomes between groups, the independent variable is the 'grouping variable'—the variable that distinguishes whether the observation for the dependent (outcome) variable is from the intervention group or the comparison group. The grouping variable is an indicator of receipt of the intervention. The possibility of confounding exists when statistically significant differences in descriptive or demographic characteristics exist between groups. Statistical testing for confounding between groups uses the grouping variable as the independent variable and the variables for descriptive or demographic characteristics as the dependent variable.

In Table 8.1, there are statistically significant differences in certain descriptive characteristics between the intervention group and the comparison group that may impact the comparison of outcome measures between the two groups. The intervention group has a significantly higher percentage of women (79.8% vs. 72.8%); of patients with asthma (42.3% vs. 35.8%); of patients with a neurological condition (12.4% vs. 9.1%); and of patients with a peripheral circulatory condition (11.8% vs. 4.2%). The intervention group has a significantly lower percentage of patients with chronic obstructive pulmonary disease (COPD; 12.9% vs. 16.6%).

Because these characteristics are significantly different between groups, they could potentially affect the outcome(s) independent of the intervention itself. For instance, if one of the outcome measures in Table 8.1 was compliance with PCP visits, it is possible that—independent of the intervention—women are more likely than men to schedule and attend PCP visits. Therefore, because there are more women in the intervention group, if PCP visits are higher in the intervention group, it is possibly *not* due to the intervention itself but to the higher percentage of women.

The next step in determining whether a variable is a confounder is to test the relationship of the confounder on the dependent variable. This is done by performing the appropriate statistical test using the potential confounder as an independent variable with the same outcome/dependent variable. In the example above, if the outcome variable was number of PCP visits, an independent *t*-test would be used to determine if the two groups (men/women) have a significantly different mean number of primary care visits. If they are statistically significantly different, then gender is a confounder impacting the results of the intervention on the outcome variable.

It is important to note the difference between an "intermediate" variable and a confounding variable. An intermediate variable is one that is part of the causal relationship between the independent variable and the outcome variable. This is more commonly distinguished in research-/knowledge-generation studies as opposed to evaluation of evidence-based translation projects. An example could be seen in a hypothetical study of the effect of obesity on end-stage renal disease. An intermediate variable could be the presence of diabetes because it can result from obesity and can lead to end-stage renal disease (Fitzmaurice, 2003).

TABLE 8.2 Testing the Impact of Potential Confounders on Outcomes

Outcome	Women	Men	Statistical Test and Result
BMI, mean (SD), (95% CI)	28.5 (3.3), (28.3–28.6)	28.8 (3.1), (28.5–29.1)	Independent *T*-Test $p = 0.029$
BMI ≥ 25, %, (95% CI)	85.5%, (83.6%–87.3%)	92.7%, (90.2%–95.2%)	Chi-Square $p = 0.000$

BMI, body mass index; CI, confidence interval; SD, standard deviation.

Using the example in Table 8.1, the potential confounder of gender is tested on the outcomes of mean body mass index (BMI) and the indicator of whether the BMI value is equal to or greater than 25 (indicator of overweight). Table 8.2 shows the results of this analysis: The mean BMI is lower for women (28.5) than for men (28.8), and a lower percentage of women have a BMI equal to or greater than 25 than men (85.5% vs. 92.7%) with $p < .05$ for both comparisons. This evaluation shows that gender has an impact on the outcome of BMI. Notice that the 95% CIs are reported for each point estimate.

PERFORMING BIVARIATE STATISTICAL TESTING OF OUTCOME MEASURES

After describing the population or events and any subgroupings and having determined whether confounding might exist, the next step is to perform bivariate statistical testing of each outcome measure. The appropriate bivariate statistic for each outcome was decided upon in the data analysis plan. However, after exploring the data and concluding whether there are violations to the assumptions of the planned bivariate test, adjustments may need to be made to the plan at this point. For instance, Tables 7.7, 7.8, and 7.9 and Figure 7.12 in Chapter 7 show the highly skewed distribution for cost data. At this point, the decision might be made to categorize cost data into meaningful categories and analyze the outcome as a categorical variable. Alternatively, a nonparametric statistical test may be used to evaluate the skewed data. Consulting with a statistician could also be warranted, if the desire is to keep the data as a continuous variable and use a more sophisticated statistical technique for handling the nonnormal distribution.

It is important to keep in mind that the final decisions about analyzing data that are made after being informed by exploratory data analysis (EDA) are as much an art as a science. There are multiple options for handling unexpected distributions and outliers in the data and each must be weighed carefully. This determination should be made in consultation with project stakeholders and a statistician. The most essential aspect of this conclusion is being able to ground the justification in clinical evidence and statistical science.

The example in Table 8.3 is a continuation of those in Tables 8.1 and 8.2. It shows the results of the bivariate analysis of the independent variable of group (intervention or comparison) and the dependent variables of BMI and BMI equal to or greater than 25. Compared to the intervention group, the comparison group

TABLE 8.3 Bivariate Testing of Outcomes

Outcome	Intervention	Comparison	Statistical Test and Result
BMI, mean (SD), (95% CI)	28.4 (3.3), (28.2–28.6)	28.7 (3.2), (28.5–28.9)	Independent *T*-Test $p = 0.106$
BMI ≥ 25, %, (95% CI)	86.5%, (84.3%–88.7%)	87.9%, (85.7%–90.2%)	Chi-Square $p = 0.357$

BMI, body mass index; CI, confidence interval; SD, standard deviation.

has a higher mean BMI (28.7 vs. 28.4) and a higher percentage of patients with a BMI equal to or greater than 25 (87.9% vs. 86.5%); however, these results are not statistically significant.

PERFORMING MULTIVARIATE TESTING OF OUTCOMES

Once it has been ascertained that the relationship between the independent and dependent variables is affected by a confounding variable, the next step is to use multivariate testing of outcomes. By doing this, a conclusion can be reached about the impact of more than one independent variable on the outcome variable. Two common types of multivariate tests are multiple linear regression and multiple logistic regression—methods covered in this chapter.

Multiple Linear Regression

Multiple linear regression is a technique used to create a model that quantifies the relationship of each of the independent variables (measured at the same time and in consideration of each other) on the dependent variable. The dependent variable must be continuous at the interval or ratio level but the independent variables can be continuous, dichotomous, or categorical. Linear regression models require certain assumptions that, when not met, can lead to inefficient or biased results. The assumptions of linear regression and other recommended guidelines are as follows:

- In order to be confident in results, there must be a large enough sample size to support each of the independent variables. A very general guideline is a minimum of 15 observations per each independent variable; nevertheless, some estimates are as high as 40 observations per independent variable. If the dependent variable is skewed, more observations are needed.
- There should not be a strong correlation between independent variables (multicollinearity). If multicollinearity exists, one independent variable could mask the effect of the other on the dependent variable; or both could look insignificant, whereas alone each could demonstrate a significant relationship with the outcome. A correlation coefficient of 0.7 between independent variables or higher suggests that multicollinearity could be an issue. Further testing is needed for confirmation. Additionally, one independent variable should not be a subset of

another independent variable (singularity). In the case of multicollinearity, one variable could be removed or a combined variable could be created from the two correlated independent variables.

- Linear regression models produce what are called "residuals." These are data points that represent the difference between the obtained and predicted outcome variable scores. The residuals should be normally distributed with an expected mean of zero; have a straight-line relationship with predicted outcome scores; be independent of each other; and have the same variance around the predicted outcome scores (Pallant, 2013).

The linear regression procedure produces a model that can be expressed in a mathematical equation. With linear regression, the values for certain components of the equation can be used to describe the impact of independent variables on the outcome/dependent variable. To illustrate, in determining the effect of a prenatal intervention for high-risk pregnancies on the outcome of birth weight, it was decided that gestational age also impacted birth weight. After running linear regression with 'birth weight' (in grams) as the outcome and 'group' (0 = comparison, 1 = intervention)

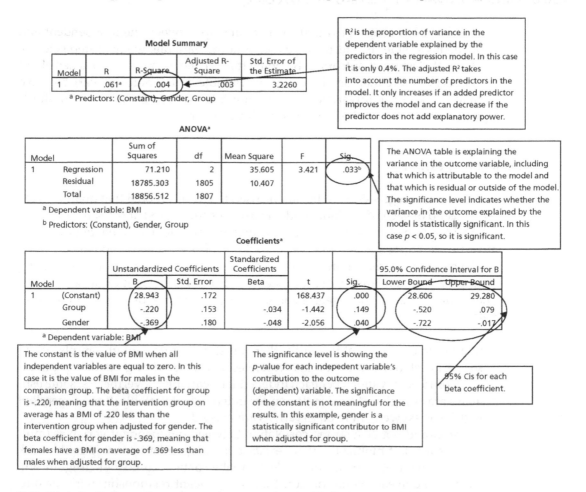

FIGURE 8.6　Selected annotated output from the linear regression model.

ANOVA, analysis of variance; BMI, body mass index; CIs, confidence intervals.
Source: Pallant (2013).

Output obtained using IBM SPSS (2012).

and 'gestational age' (in weeks) as independent variables, the following model was developed and expressed by the equation:

$$\text{birth weight} = 2{,}635 + (500 \times \text{group}) + (10.3 \times \text{gestational age})$$

In this model, the value of 2,635 is a constant and represents the birth weight when the values of all other variables (group and gestational age) are equal to zero. However, it is difficult to interpret the constant when there are independent variables that do not have a range that realistically reaches zero (as is the case with gestational age). The constant is used when determining the value of birth weight, given certain values for each of the independent variables; in this case, that is for a certain group assignment and certain gestational age. The values of 500 and 10.3 are called beta coefficients; in order to interpret them, it is important to understand the possible values and coding of those values for each independent variable. Because group is coded as 1 = intervention and 0 = group, the beta coefficient of 500 is interpreted

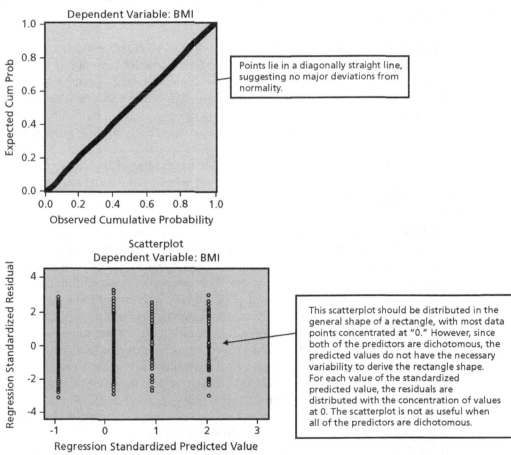

FIGURE 8.7   Selected annotated output from the linear regression model.

BMI, body mass index; P-P plot, probability-probability plot.
Source: Pallant (2013).
Output obtained using IBM SPSS (2012).

as "holding gestational age constant, birth weight is 500 grams higher, on average, for women in the intervention group than in the comparison group." The value of 10.3 is interpreted as "for every 1-week increase in gestational age, the expected birth weight increases by 10.3 grams," holding group constant. The expected birth weight for the child of a woman in the intervention group with a gestational age of 40 would be equal to $2,635 + (500 \times 1) + (10.3 \times 40) = 3,547$ grams.

Continuing with the example in Figures 8.1 through 8.5, linear regression is used to determine whether consideration of gender in the relationship between the intervention and BMI changes the impact of the intervention on BMI. To run linear regression in SPSS, choose **Analyze → Regression → Linear**. Next, **Method** should be picked as 'Enter'; selected **Statistics** include 'Estimates,' 'Confidence Intervals,' 'Model Fit,' 'Descriptives,' 'Part and partial correlations,' and 'Collinearity diagnositics'; selected **Plots** include '*ZRESID' in the 'Y' box and '*ZPPRED' in the 'X' box, and 'Normal probability plot' under 'Standard Residual Plots' (Pallant, 2013). Figure 8.6 and Figure 8.7 annotate selected portions of the SPSS output for the linear regression model.

Multiple Logistic Regression

Multiple logistic regression is also a method used to create a model that quantifies the relationship of each of the independent variables (measured at the same time and in consideration of each other) on the dependent variable. As opposed to linear regression, in logistic regression the dependent variable is dichotomous (other types of logistic models exist for dependent variables with more than two categories). The independent variables are usually dichotomous, categorical, or ordinal and can also be continuous.

There are also a few guiding principles for the use of logistic regression. As in linear regression, it is important to explore whether the independent variables are highly correlated with each other (a correlation coefficient of 0.7 or higher may be too high). The results of logistic regression are highly sensitive to the effects of multicollinearity and outliers, so care must be taken in reducing these effects (Pallant, 2013). Additionally, when using logistic regression it is important to have a sample size that is large enough so that each category within the independent variables is not lacking in observations. For example, if one of the independent variables is race and a small amount of people fall into one of the race categories, this poses a problem in producing results. Logistic regression is not based on a normal distribution; therefore, it does not require many of the same assumptions as linear regression—except that the observations be independent (Pallant, 2013).

For better interpretation, categorical variables and ordinal variables can be changed into "dummy variables" by creating separate variables that are yes/ no indicators for each value of the original categorical variable. For instance, the categorical variable 'bed type' that has values of 'medical,' 'surgical,' 'obstetrics,' etc. would be changed into three individual variables of 'medical,' 'surgical,' and 'obstetrics' with values of '1' = yes, '0' = no for each of the variables. For interpretability, all dichotomous variables are coded as '1,' '0,' and all categorical and ordinal variables (without dummy coding) have at least one category that is coded as '0' and ordered numbering for subsequent categories (e.g., '0,' '1,' '2,' '3,' etc.). The category coded as '0' is called the reference category and represents the classification to which all other categories are compared. With a string of dummy variables, one value is omitted and thus is the reference category.

The logistic regression model can also be expressed in a mathematical formula. However, with logistic regression, exponentiated beta coefficients are used to interpret the impact of independent variables. The coefficients from SPSS output are provided as a "B" beta coefficient and an "Exp(B)" exponentiated beta coefficient. Interpreting the impact of each individual independent variable on the dependent variable, the Exp(B) value that is equal to the odds ratio is used (UCLA: Statistical Consulting Group, 2013). The odds ratio is the estimated difference in the odds of the dependent variable for a 1-unit increase in the value of the independent variable. In other words, for every 1-unit increase in the independent variable, the odds of the dependent variable occurring changes by a factor of the odds ratio. (Odds are defined as the probability that an event occurs divided by the probability that an event does *not* occur.) An odds ratio of 1 means that the independent variable does not affect the odds of the dependent variable (in other words, the odds are equivalent between groups); an odds ratio of greater than 1 is associated with higher odds of the dependent variable; and an odds ratio of less than 1 is associated with lower odds of the dependent variable (Szumilas, 2010).

In this example, the dependent variable in the linear regression formula is changed to 'birth weight > 2,700' (1 = yes and 0 = no); and the independent variables are entered as "group" (0 = comparison, 1 = intervention) and "gestational age category" (0 = < 37 weeks, 1 = ≥ 37 weeks). Notice that the reference group (the group with the value of 0) for gestational age is set at the value that is considered a lower than normal gestational age. This is important for interpreting results. The following Exp(B) (odds ratio) coefficients are output by the SPSS logistic regression function:

- Exp(B) for group = 1.87
- Exp(B) for gestational age category = 1.27

Using the exponentiated beta coefficients for describing the impact of individual independent variables, it is best to discuss this impact in terms of odds and predicted probabilities. In this statistical logistic model, the odds of having a baby with a birth weight over 2,700 grams are 1.87 times (or 87%) greater for a woman in the intervention group than in the comparison group, adjusting for gestational age. This relationship can also be expressed in terms of the probability of having a baby with a birth weight over 2,700 grams using the following formula (Fleiss, 1981):

$$\text{odds ratio} / 1 + \text{odds ratio}$$

The predicted probability for a woman in the intervention group of having a baby with a birth weight greater than 2,700 grams is 1.87/1 + 1.87 = 0.65. The probability for a woman in the intervention group of having a baby with a birth weight greater than 2,700 grams is 65%, adjusted for gestational age.

Continuing with the example in Figures 8.1 through 8.7, logistic regression is applied to the outcome of BMI equal to or greater than 25 to determine if consideration of gender in the relationship between the intervention and BMI changes the impact of the intervention on BMI. To run logistic regression in SPSS, select **Analyze → Regression → Binary Logistic**. Choose the appropriate dependent and independent variable(s). Next, **Method** should be selected as 'Enter'; selected **Options** include 'Classification Plots,' 'Hosmer-Lemeshow Goodness of Fit,' and 'CI for Exp(B)' (Pallant, 2013). Figure 8.8 annotates selected portions of the SPSS output for the logistic regression model.

Block 0: Beginning Block

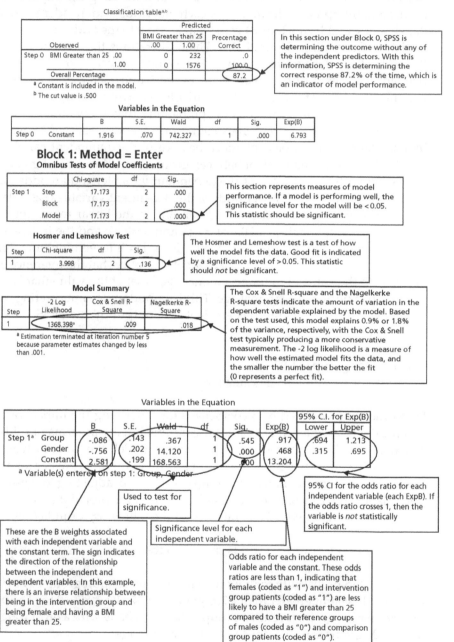

Classification table[a,b]

		Predicted		
		BMI Greater than 25		Precentage Correct
Observed		.00	1.00	
Step 0 BMI Greater than 25 .00		0	232	.0
1.00		0	1576	100.0
Overall Percentage				87.2

[a] Constant is included in the model.
[b] The cut value is .500

In this section under Block 0, SPSS is determining the outcome without any of the independent predictors. With this information, SPSS is determining the correct response 87.2% of the time, which is an indicator of model performance.

Variables in the Equation

		B	S.E.	Wald	df	Sig.	Exp(B)
Step 0	Constant	1.916	.070	742.327	1	.000	6.793

Block 1: Method = Enter
Omnibus Tests of Model Coefficients

		Chi-square	df	Sig.
Step 1	Step	17.173	2	.000
	Block	17.173	2	.000
	Model	17.173	2	.000

This section represents measures of model performance. If a model is performing well, the significance level for the model will be < 0.05. This statistic should be significant.

Hosmer and Lemeshow Test

Step	Chi-square	df	Sig.
1	3.998	2	.136

The Hosmer and Lemeshow test is a test of how well the model fits the data. Good fit is indicated by a significance level of > 0.05. This statistic should *not* be significant.

Model Summary

Step	-2 Log Likelihood	Cox & Snell R-Square	Nagelkerke R-Square
1	1368.398[a]	.009	.018

[a] Estimation terminated at iteration number 5 because parameter estimates changed by less than .001.

The Cox & Snell R-square and the Nagelkerke R-square tests indicate the amount of variation in the dependent variable explained by the model. Based on the test used, this model explains 0.9% or 1.8% of the variance, respectively, with the Cox & Snell test typically producing a more conservative measurement. The -2 log likelihood is a measure of how well the estimated model fits the data, and the smaller the number the better the fit (0 represents a perfect fit).

Variables in the Equation

		B	S.E.	Wald	df	Sig.	Exp(B)	95% C.I. for Exp(B)	
								Lower	Upper
Step 1[a]	Group	-.086	.143	.367	1	.545	.917	.694	1.213
	Gender	-.756	.202	14.120	1	.000	.468	.315	.695
	Constant	2.581	.199	168.563	1	.000	13.204		

[a] Variable(s) entered on step 1: Group, Gender.

Used to test for significance.

These are the B weights associated with each independent variable and the constant term. The sign indicates the direction of the relationship between the independent and dependent variables. In this example, there is an inverse relationship between being in the intervention group and being female and having a BMI greater than 25.

Significance level for each independent variable.

95% CI for the odds ratio for each independent variable (each ExpB). If the odds ratio crosses 1, then the variable is *not* statistically significant.

Odds ratio for each independent variable and the constant. These odds ratios are less than 1, indicating that females (coded as "1") and intervention group patients (coded as "1") are less likely to have a BMI greater than 25 compared to their reference groups of males (coded as "0") and comparison group patients (coded as "0").

FIGURE 8.8   Selected annotated output from the logistic regression model.

BMI, body mass index; CI, confidence interval; SE = standard error.
Source: Pallant (2013).
Output obtained using IBM SPSS (2012).

OTHER CONSIDERATIONS WHEN MEASURING OUTCOMES

This chapter covers methods for bivariate and multivariate testing of outcomes using the most common statistical procedures. Here and in Chapter 7, data are explored to determine whether the distributions meet assumptions that are necessary for these tests. Some suggestions are given about how to handle data for outcome measurement when they do not meet the assumptions. This section broadly introduces some of the alternatives to the described statistical testing of outcomes when data do not meet the necessary assumptions. It is important to consult with a statistician when considering the options.

Nonparametric Testing

Chapter 2 reviews the types of nonparametric statistical tests and their appropriate use. Nonparametric tests do not depend on the assumption of normality of the data. Instead, these tests utilize ranking of the data and rely on the median as opposed to the mean. These methods are often employed when data do not meet the normality assumptions needed for parametric testing or when the sample size is too small. Nonparametric techniques are considered to be less powerful and less flexible than parametric tests. This should be taken into account when deciding to use them (Keller & Kelvin, 2013).

Complex Statistical Models

Complex statistical models can be developed to measure the outcomes between groups when data do not meet the assumptions for the more common tests. For instance, in Chapter 6 the special case of cost data is described with a distribution of many values at zero and a strongly positive skew. A special type of statistical model, called a "two-part model," can be designed to measure outcomes. Using this technique, two statistical models are created that use all the data separated into zero costs and positive costs. These two models are then considered together when determining overall cost differences (Robinson, Zeger, & Forrest, 2006).

In addition to the reasons previously mentioned for seeking alternative statistical models, there are some commonly seen data distributions that warrant consideration of complex statistical models. One of these distributions is the case of a rare outcome—for example, death. Rare outcomes can be a problem when measuring results such as readmissions that have a low incidence. Rare events can be even more challenging when sample sizes are small (fewer than 100 patients). Depending on the sample size, with rare outcomes a nonparametric model or a complex statistical model may be considered.

Complex statistical models may also be contemplated when measuring results in longitudinal data with multiple time-incremented observations per person. Examples of these data include minute-by-minute observations of fetal heart rate, time-stamped call light occurrences, and monthly observations of quality or cost outcomes over multiple years. In these situations, it may be very important to have the outcomes analysis be informed by all data points—instead of altering the data to meet the requirements of one of the more commonly understood bivariate or multivariate statistical tests, which require that observations be independent. For example, patterns of call lights that identify determinants of outcomes such as time of day, day of week, staff available, etc. can be ascertained from using all detailed call light data. These might not be discerned if data were transformed to meet the requirements of a commonly used statistical test.

SUMMARY

Measurement of successful outcomes is the final step in the journey of clinical data management (CDM). It is undertaken with a clear understanding of each individual variable that was accomplished during EDA. The methods for statistically testing outcomes are taken from the data analysis plan with consideration of findings from EDA. Decisions about methods utilized to test outcomes are grounded equally in the science of statistics and in the science of clinical evidence. The final decision about how to measure results is both an art and a science.

REFERENCES

Centers for Medicare and Medicaid Services. (2013, July 10). CMS.Gov. *Medicare Claims Synthetic Public Use Files (SynPUFs)*. Retrieved August 13, 2013, from http://www.cms.gov/Research-Statistics-Data-and-Systems/Statistics-Trends-and-Reports/SynPUFs/

Fitzmaurice, G. (2003). Confused by confounding? *Nutrition, 19*(2), 189–191.

Fleiss, J. L. (1981). Sampling method I: Naturalistic or cross-sectional studies. In J. L. Fleiss (Ed.), *Statistical methods for rates and proportions* (pp. 65–66). New York, NY: Wiley.

IBM. (2012). *IBM SPSS Statistics for Windows, version 21.0*. Armonk, NY: Author.

Keller, S. B. P., & Kelvin, E. (2013). *Munro's statistical methods for healthcare research* (6th ed.). Philadelphia, PA: Lippincott Williams & Wilkins.

Nightengale, F. (1863). *Notes on hospitals*. London, UK: Saville and Edwards Printers. Retrieved from https://archive.org/details/notesonhospital01nighgoog

Pallant, J. (2013). *SPSS survival manual*. New York, NY: McGraw-Hill.

Robinson, J. W., Zeger, S. L., & Forrest, C. B. (2006). A hierarchical multivariate two-part model for profiling providers' effects on health care charges. *Journal of the American Statistical Association, 101*(475), 911–923.

Szumilas, M. (2010). Explaining odds ratios. *Journal of the Canadian Academy of Child and Adolescent Psychiatry, 19*(3), 227–229.

UCLA: Statistical Consulting Group. (2013). *Understanding odds ratios in binary logistic regression*. Retrieved September 6, 2013, from http://www.ats.ucla.edu/stat/stata/library/odds_ratio_logistic.htm

CASE STUDY

CASE STUDY EXAMPLE: OUTCOMES DATA ANALYSIS (ODA)

DESCRIPTION OF CHARACTERISTICS FOR INTERVENTION AND COMPARISON GROUPS WITHIN THE OLDER COMMUNITY-DWELLING PATIENTS WITH DIABETES

The following table shows the differences in means and proportions for the demographic characteristics, morbidity level, and certain illness prevalence between the intervention group and the comparison group. As noted previously, the intervention group has a higher percentage of patients in the high risk and very high risk morbidity categories, when combining the two groups, compared to the comparison group (74.0% vs. 64.7%, $p < .05$). The prevalence of distinct illnesses is similar between both groups except for cancer—where the intervention group has a rate of 9.1% and the comparison group has a rate of 17.4% ($p < .05$), and diabetic retinopathy—where the intervention group has a rate of 12.5% and the comparison group has a rate of 6.5%.

Characteristic	Intervention	Comparison	Statistic Used for Comparison	Statistical Significance
Number in group	208	184	N/A	N/A
Age mean (range)	74.4 (65–100)	74.9 (65–96)	Independent t-test	Not significant
% Women	44.0%	38.9%	Chi-square	Not significant
Race				
% White	43.3%	46.2%		
% Black	51.9%	52.7%	Chi-square	Not significant
% Hispanic	4.8%	1.1%		
Morbidity level				
% Low risk	0.5%	2.2%	Chi-square	$p < .05$, significant (Note, assumptions for chi-square are not met when broken down into these categories. The chi-square test is significant when the dichotomizing variable and assumptions are met.)

(continued)

(continued)

Characteristic	Intervention	Comparison	Statistic Used for Comparison	Statistical Significance
% Moderate risk	25.5%	33.2%		
% High risk	39.4%	43.5%		
% Very high risk	34.6%	21.2%		
% AMI	3.4%	3.8%	Chi-square	Not significant
% Anxiety/neurosis	5.8%	10.3%	Chi-square	Not significant
% Asthma	2.9%	3.3%	Chi-square	Not significant
% Blindness	1.0%	0.5%	Chi-square	Not significant
% Cancer	9.1%	17.4%	Chi-square	$p < .05$, significant
% Cardiac arrest	1.0%	1.1%	Chi-square	Not significant
% Cardiomyopathy	2.4%	1.1%	Chi-square	Not significant
% Cerebrovascular disease	13.0%	14.7%	Chi-square	Not significant
% Chronic liver disease	0.5%	0.5%	Chi-square	Not significant
% Chronic pancreatitis	1.0%	0.5%	Chi-square	Not significant
% Chronic renal failure	10.1%	9.2%	Chi-square	Not significant
% Chronic skin ulcer	3.4%	2.2%	Chi-square	Not significant
% Congestive heart failure	11.1%	10.9%	Chi-square	Not significant
% Degenerative joint disease	38.0%	31.0%	Chi-square	Not significant
% Dementia/delirium	5.8%	6.0%	Chi-square	Not significant
% Depression	8.2%	10.9%	Chi-square	Not significant
% Diabetic retinopathy	12.5%	6.5%	Chi-square	$p < .05$, significant
% Disorder of lipoid metabolism	75.0%	75.0%	Chi-square	Not significant
% Emphysema/chronic bronchitis/COPD	6.7%	11.4%	Chi-square	Not significant
% Generalized atherosclerosis	27.9%	23.4%	Chi-square	Not significant

(continued)

(continued)

Characteristic	Intervention	Comparison	Statistic Used for Comparison	Statistical Significance
% Glaucoma	24.5%	29.3%	Chi-square	Not significant
% Hypertension	79.3%	85.3%	Chi-square	Not significant
% Ischemic heart disease	25.0%	28.8%	Chi-square	Not significant
% Obesity	21.6%	15.2%	Chi-square	Not significant
% Ophthalmic signs/ symptoms	2.4%	1.1%	Chi-square	Not significant
% Parkinson's disease	1.4%	1.6%	Chi-square	Not significant
% Peripheral neuropathy	13.5%	15.2%	Chi-square	Not significant
% Tobacco use	4.3%	4.3%	Chi-square	Not significant
% Transplant	0.5%	0.5%	Chi-square	Not significant

AMI, acute myocardial infarction; COPD, chronic obstructive pulmonary disease; N/A, not applicable.

RECOGNIZING POSSIBLE CONFOUNDING IN THE OLDER COMMUNITY-DWELLING PATIENTS WITH DIABETES

Thoughtful review of the exploratory analysis for this population indicates that morbidity level is a potential confounder of the relationship between the intervention and the outcomes. There are statistically significant different rates of cancer and diabetic retinopathy between the two groups; however, this variable was not tested as a confounder because of the problem of singularity, since presence of cancer and diabetic retinopathy are both considered in the determination of morbidity level. In order to ascertain if these outcomes are significantly different between the intervention group and the comparison group, statistical testing of morbidity level between groups is warranted. Because the distribution of morbidity level is not amenable to means testing and there is a higher percentage of high risk and very high risk morbidity levels in the intervention group compared to the comparison group, the morbidity level variable is dichotomized into two categories—one for "high risk" and "very high risk" and the second for "moderate risk" and "low risk." The moderate risk/low risk group is coded as "0" and the high risk/very high risk group is coded as "1." (It is important to code all dichotomous variables as 1, 0, as mentioned previously.)

The following SPSS output shows that the percentage of those with high morbidity is higher in the intervention group than in the comparison group (74.0% vs. 64.7%). The assumptions for chi-square are met with 0% of cells having an expected count of < 5. The *p* value of .044 indicates that the distribution of patients with high morbidity within the intervention group and the comparison group is significantly different. It is therefore possible that morbidity level is a confounder in the relationship between receiving the intervention and outcomes. This is tested next.

Grouping Within the Population *Morbidity Level Dichotomized Crosstabulation			Morbidity Level Dichotomized		
			Low Morbidity	High Morbidity	Total
Group within the population	Comparison	Count	65	119	184
		% within grouping within the population	35.3%	64.7%	100.0%
		% within morbidity level dichotomized	54.6%	43.6%	46.9%
	Intervention	Count	54	154	208
		% within grouping within the population	26.0%	74.0%	100.0%
		% within morbidity level dichotomized	45.4%	56.4%	53.1%
Total		Count	119	273	392
		% within grouping within the population	30.4%	69.6%	100.0%
		% within morbidity level dichotomized	100.0%	100.0%	100.0%

Chi-Square Tests					
	Value	df	Asymp. Sig. (2-sided)	Exact Sig. (2-sided)	Exact Sig. (1-sided)
Pearson chi-square	4.500[a]	1	.044		
Continuity correction[b]	3.619	1	.057		
Likelihood ratio	4.048	1	.044		
Fisher's exact test				.048	.029
Linear-by-linear association	4.039	1	.044		
No. of valid cases	392				

[a] 0 cells (0.0%) have expected count less than 5. The minimum expected count is 55.86. [b] Computed only for a 2 x 2 table.

The following table shows the results of the evaluation of whether having high morbidity versus low morbidity impacts measures of hemoglobin A1C (HbA1C) or admissions in the older community-dwelling patients with diabetes population. Compared to the low morbidity group, the high morbidity group has a higher mean pre-HbA1C to post-HbA1C increase (low = 0.09 vs. high = 0.41), but that difference is not statistically significant. Those in the high morbidity group have an increase of 0.07 from preadmissions to post-admissions compared to the low morbidity group with a decrease of 0.29 from preadmissions to postadmissions. These differences are statistically meaningful ($p = .001$). Additionally, 36% of the high morbidity group have a postperiod admission compared to 5% of the low morbidity group ($p = .000$). Morbidity is having an impact on admission-related outcomes but not on HbA1C-related outcomes.

Morbidity Group	Difference in Pre-HbA1C to Post-HbA1C	Statistical Test and Result	Difference in Preadmissions to Post-admissions	Statistical Test and Result	Presence of an Admission in the Postperiod	Statistical Test and Result
High morbidity	Mean (SD), (95% CI) 0.41 (1.94), (0.18–0.64)	Independent t-test $p = .139$	Mean (SD), (95% CI) 0.07 (1.32), (−0.08–0.23)	Independent t-test $p = .001$ (equal variances not assumed)	% High morbidity, (95% CI) 36.0%, (31.0%–42.0%)	Chi-square $p = .000$
Low morbidity	Mean (SD), (95% CI) 0.09 (1.93), (−0.26–0.44)		Mean (SD), (95% CI) −0.29 (0.86), (−0.45–[−0.14])		% Low morbidity, (95% CI) 5.0%, (1.0%–9.0%)	

CI, confidence interval; HbA1C, hemoglobin A1C; SD, standard deviation.

RECOGNIZING POSSIBLE CONFOUNDING IN INPATIENT ADMISSIONS

Testing for confounding is not applicable in the analysis of inpatient admissions because the readmissions outcome is descriptive and there is no comparison group.

OUTCOMES DETERMINATION FOR OLDER COMMUNITY-DWELLING PATIENTS WITH DIABETES

- HbA1C value 6 months following the start of the intervention
  - Due to the skewed distribution of the data for HbA1C, it was decided to examine the results statistically using nonparametric tests. The Mann-Whitney U (nonparametric tests are found under **Analyze → Nonparametric Tests** in SPSS) test is assessed. The table that follows shows the intervention group has a lower mean HbA1C in the postperiod contrasted with the comparison group (7.86 vs. 8.30). The differences in HbA1C are statistically significant using the Mann-Whitney U nonparametric rank test ($p = .009$).

Outcome	Intervention	Comparison	Statistical Test and Result
HbA1C, mean (SD), (95% CI) median	7.86 (1.54), (7.69, 8.03) 7.70	8.30 (1.41), (8.10, 8.50) 7.70	Mann-Whitney U test $p = .009$

CI, confidence interval; HbA1C, hemoglobin A1C; SD, standard deviation.

- Difference in HbA1C values from preintervention to postintervention
  - An independent *t*-test is used to analyze the difference between the intervention and comparison groups in the change in HbA1C values from preintervention to postintervention. The intervention group has a mean decrease of 0.09 in the HbA1C value from preintervention to postintervention, whereas the comparison group has a mean increase of 0.76 ($p < .001$). These results are statistically significant.

Outcome	Intervention	Comparison	Statistical Test and Result
HbA1C, mean (SD), (95% CI)	−0.09 (1.85), (−0.34, 0.17)	0.76 (1.95), (0.47, 1.04)	Independent *t*-test $p < .001$

CI, confidence interval; HbA1C, hemoglobin A1C; SD, standard deviation.

- Number of admissions in the postperiod
  - Due to the extremely skewed distribution of the data for admissions, it was decided to examine the results of statistical analysis using the Mann-Whitney U nonparametric test. The following table shows that the intervention group has a lower mean number of admissions in the postperiod compared to the comparison group (0.29 vs. 0.55). The differences in number of admissions are statistically significant utilizing the Mann-Whitney U nonparametric rank test ($p = .001$).

Outcome	Intervention	Comparison	Statistical Test and Result
No. of admissions, mean (SD), (95% CI) median	0.29 (0.68), (0.20, 0.38) 0.00	0.55 (0.91), (0.42, 0.69) 0.00	Mann-Whitney U test $p = .001$

CI, confidence interval; SD, standard deviation.

- Difference in number of admissions from preintervention to postintervention
  - An independent *t*-test is employed to examine the difference between the intervention and comparison groups in the change in number of admissions from preintervention to postintervention. The intervention group has a mean decrease of 0.14 admissions from preintervention to postintervention, whereas the comparison group has a mean increase of 0.08; however, these results are not statistically significant ($p = .075$).

Outcome	Intervention	Comparison	Statistical Test and Result
Difference in no. of admissions, mean (SD), (95% CI)	−0.14, (−0.26, 0.03)	0.08 (1.53), (−0.14, 0.30)	Independent *t*-test $p = .075$

CI, confidence interval; SD, standard deviation.

- Indicator of an admission in the postperiod
  - A chi-square test is used to test the difference between the intervention and comparison groups in the occurrence of an admission in the postperiod. Within the intervention group, 19.7% of patients have an admission, whereas 34.8% of those in the comparison group have an admission. These results are significant ($p = .001$).

Outcome	Intervention	Comparison	Statistical Test and Result
Indicator of an admission, %, (95% CI)	19.7%, (14.3%, 25.2%)	34.8% (27.8%, 44.7%)	Chi-square test $p = .001$

CI, confidence interval.

OUTCOMES DETERMINATION FOR THE INPATIENT ADMISSIONS GROUP OF EVENTS

No further analysis is necessary beyond that carried out in the EDA in Chapter 7.

OUTCOMES DETERMINATION WITH ADJUSTMENT FOR CONFOUNDING FOR OLDER COMMUNITY-DWELLING PATIENTS WITH DIABETES

- Adjustment for confounding by 'morbidity level' is done for the following outcomes:
  - Difference in pre-HbA1C to post-HbA1C—linear regression
  - Difference in number of preadmissions to postadmissions—linear regression
  - Occurrence of an admission in the postperiod—logistic regression

The outcomes of 'HbA1C value in the postperiod' and '# of admissions in the postperiod' do not meet the assumptions necessary for linear regression. Nonparametric determination of statistical significance is reported for these results.

	Difference in Pre-HbA1C to Post-HbA1C Mean Change in Outcome With 1-Unit Increase in Independent Variable (95% CI) (p Value) R^2 for Model = 5.7%	Difference in Preadmissions to Postadmissions Mean Change in Outcome With 1-Unit Increase in Independent Variable (95% CI) (p Value) R^2 for Model = 3.1%	Occurrence of an Admission in the Postperiod Odds Ratio (95% CI) (p Value) Hosmer-Lemeshow p Value = .365
Group (1 = intervention, 0 = comparison)	-0.88 (-1.26, -0.51) ($p < .001$)	-0.26 (-0.50, -0.02) ($p = .031$)	0.36 (0.21, 0.57) ($p < .001$)
Morbidity level (1 = high, 0 = low)	0.41 (0.00, 0.82) ($p = .048$)	0.40 (0.14, 0.66) ($p = .003$)	13.1 (5.46, 31.28) ($p < .001$)

CI, confidence interval; HbA1C, hemoglobin A1C; R^2, coefficient of determination.

- Difference in pre-HbA1C to post-HbA1C—linear regression
  - The change in HbA1C values is on average 0.88 points lower for those in the intervention group versus the comparison group, adjusting for morbidity level ($p < .001$) (a negative difference indicates a better result for the intervention group).
- Difference in number of preadmissions to postadmissions—linear regression
  - The difference in the number of admissions is on average 0.26 lower per year for those in the intervention group versus the comparison group, adjusting for morbidity level ($p = .031$).
- Occurrence of an admission in the postperiod—logistic regression
  - The odds of having an admission are 0.36 times (or 64% less) for those in the intervention group versus the comparison group, adjusting for morbidity level ($p < .001$).

CHAPTER 9

Summarizing the Results of the Project Evaluation

MARTHA L. SYLVIA

This chapter addresses the components of reporting the results of the evaluation of the Doctor of Nursing Practice (DNP) project. The focus here is on documentation of quantitative results. Therefore, detailing of the overall project or of qualitative or descriptive results is not included. Reporting of results is done within a defined structure; however, the content within that structure and the choice of format and mechanisms for delivery are chosen based on the primary interest of the target audience. Hence, this chapter describes the basic elements that need to be compiled for the recording of outcomes. Variation is expected in the actual communication and presentation of this information, based on the targeted audience and message.

LEARNING OBJECTIVES

After reading this chapter, the DNP should be able to:

- Create flow diagrams
- Describe limitations within the data management process that may impact results
- Design oral and written presentations of outcomes that focus on audience/stakeholder interests
- Use a defined structure to report the quantitative results of DNP project outcomes

REPORTING RESULTS

The structure for reporting of results falls under the following headings and subheadings:

- Data management plan
  - Description of population or events
  - Power analysis and sample size determination
  - Explanation of aims, outcomes, measures, and statistics

- Flow of participants/events
- Data collection
- Data governance
- Data cleansing and manipulation
- Exploratory data analysis (EDA) results
- Outcomes data analysis (ODA) results
- Summary of results
- Data limitations

Summarizing the Data Management Plan

The first step in reporting the results of the project evaluation is to describe key elements of the original plan for analysis. This is similar to the description of methods in a research study. The initial detailing should cover the unit(s) of analyses (population and/or events), including the inclusion and exclusion criteria and the criteria for assignment to the intervention group or comparison group.

Next, a summary of the power analysis is provided. Key elements to include in this description are:

- An explanation of the choice of measure for power analysis
- A description of the expected differences in the measure, including the point estimate for the mean or proportion
- Evidence supporting this expected difference in the measure
- Choice of statistical test
- Alpha or significance level
- Power
- Method of calculation or the chosen sample size calculator
- Resulting required sample size

Flow Diagrams

Following the summary of the data management plan, a flow chart can be used to diagram the progress of individuals or events. Flow charts provide an organized method for explaining the process of identifying the population or set of events for analysis and describing any loss of numbers due to procedures that occur during the project. A structured method for creating flow charts for research was developed and revised in the Consolidated Standards of Reporting Trials (CONSORT) statement (Schulz, Altman, & Moher, 2010). This format also works well for reporting the identification and progress of a population or set of events in an evidence-translation project evaluation and is commonly referred to as a "CONSORT diagram."

The CONSORT diagram divides the flow of the progress of the population or set of events into four stages: enrollment, allocation, follow-up, and analysis (Moher, Schulz, & Altman, 2001). In each stage, the number in each grouping is provided along with a short description of the reasons for inclusion and/or attrition, resulting in a tally of the final number included in the evaluation. The enrollment stage in a translation project is the phase in which inclusion and exclusion criteria are applied. The allocation stage comes after the inclusion and exclusion criteria are applied, and the assignment of individuals or events to the intervention group or the comparison group is executed. The follow-up phase represents the time in the project when the intervention is implemented. During this stage—and usually where the unit of analysis is individuals—loss of numbers due to unforeseen circumstances can occur (e.g., patient self-removal from the intervention, loss of staff, organizational changes, etc.). The analysis phase coincides with the stage of data management when all data are collected and the EDA is under way. During this phase of EDA, any decisions to remove individuals or events from the evaluation are described in the analysis section of the CONSORT diagram. The analysis section reports the final number for analysis in each group and, if applicable, indicates whether the sample size in each group is large enough to achieve statistical power.

Figure 9.1 is an example of a CONSORT diagram used in an evidence-translation project. Templates for CONSORT diagrams are available from the CONSORT group (CONSORT Group, n.d.).

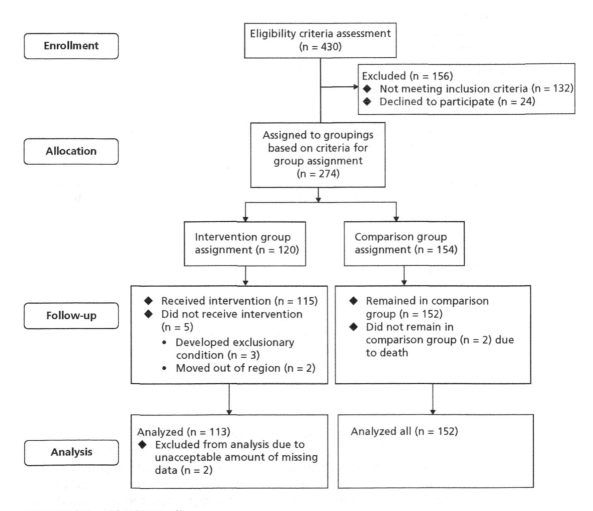

FIGURE 9.1   CONSORT diagram.
Adapted from Moher et al. (2001).

Data Collection Processes

Next, the process of data collection should be described. In this section, the data-collection methods are explained first by indicating whether primary or secondary data are collected. If primary data are collected, the data collection tool should be detailed, including any reliability and validity evidence if available. If the tool was designed specifically for this project, there should be a description of the evidence supporting the development of the tool. Additionally, the methods for administering the tool should be described. For instance: Who filled out the tool and by what means (e.g., in writing, verbal response, etc.)? What was the timing of administration of the tool? What were the circumstances under which it was completed? The methods for entering the responses or data collected from the tool into an electronic data system should also be explained. For example: Who entered the data? What software was used to enter data electronically? When were the data entered? Finally, the transfer of data between the software used for data entry and the eventual software for data analysis should be detailed.

If secondary data are collected, the source(s) of the data should be described as well as the primary reason for collecting the data. For instance, diagnoses on hospital billing data used in a translation project to detail disease conditions for a population of patients are collected primarily for the purposes of billing insurance companies for reimbursement. Describing the source of secondary data collection, it is important to provide the following where applicable:

- The circumstances under which the data are collected: Are data entered into a checklist at the patient bedside or are they entered by clinicians completing paperwork at the end of a shift? Are data collected by a telemonitoring device?
- A description of any telemonitoring devices and related software.
- The role of any person entering the data: For instance, hospitals hire coders who review charts and complete billing forms that are submitted to insurance companies.
- The role of any person generating the data: For instance, clinicians enter the information into medical charts that are used by the coders to complete the billing forms.
- The timing of the collection of the data: Are data collected once per shift, per day, or per minute?
- Any and all software used in the data collection process.

As with primary data collection, the transfer of data between the software used for data entry and the eventual software for data analysis should be described.

Data Governance

The process of data governance should be summarized in any final reporting of results. The summary includes the procedures and applications to the appropriate institutional review board (IRB) and the decisions of the IRB regarding project approval. Some IRBs have a process in place to determine whether a project does or does not require IRB application submission. If this type of procedure was followed and it was determined that the project does not require IRB approval, the criteria by which the project was determined to *not* need approval should be explained.

Regardless of whether the project requires IRB approval, the management of data security should be detailed—including the location of data storage; the processes for all transfers of data (e.g., secure e-mail, file transfer protocol [FTP], postal mail, etc.); persons who have ongoing access to the data; and the plan for archiving or destroying the data once the project and evaluation are completed.

Data Cleansing and Manipulation

Despite the fact that the data cleansing and manipulation phase of data management is one of the most lengthy and time-consuming, most audiences and key stakeholders do not have a great interest in the details of the steps necessary to create the final analysis data set. What they might be interested in are: (a) methods for handling missing data; (b) a summary of any calculations of definitions for newly derived variables, particularly those not originally defined in the analysis plan; (c) any challenges in data cleansing that require a major change in the original analysis plan; and (d) a brief description of the design of the final analysis data set.

For reference purposes, it is important to have a record of all the steps taken during this phase of data management. The rough draft of the description of these steps should already be documented in the syntax file. It is useful to have available a summary of the key decision points and actions taken during data cleansing and manipulation. This can be organized as personal notes or extra hidden slides when presenting the results, and can be referenced when related questions are asked.

Exploratory Data Analysis

The results of EDA should be summarized in a way that leads the audience into an understanding of the final results of the project evaluation. It is meaningful to describe distributions of variables and significant findings about outliers in this section. The reporting of EDA begins with the description of the population and/ or set of events with a comparison of differences on key characteristics between subgroupings. Distributions of descriptive and/or demographic variables should be detailed when factors of the pattern such as outliers or skewness lead to removal of some data points or the restructuring of key variables.

Distributions of key outcome variables should be described and include an analysis of whether the variable is appropriately distributed for the planned statistical test. After detailing key outcome variables, any findings that indicate potential confounding should be described. The EDA section of the results should conclude with a summary statement of the findings during EDA and any decision making about variables and measurement that results in a change to the original analysis plan. For instance, the presence of outliers may lead to the removal of data points, or the distribution of data points for certain variables may lead to a decision to change the structure of the variable (e.g., from continuous to dichotomous).

The choice of display for the EDA summary is dependent on the audience and the method of delivery of the results (e.g., written or oral). It is best to use easy-to-interpret tables and graphs. For this section, graphs should be limited to those that display distributions of continuous variables. Boxplots and histograms are most easily understood by a wide variety of audiences. Keep in mind that whereas more detailed plots such as stem-and-leaf plots provide a great deal of information that is useful in analyzing the data, it is better to use graphics that take the least amount of explaining to get the point across when presenting the data. If in doubt, it is always helpful to ask someone who is unfamiliar with the data to give feedback on interpretability of graphics in written and presentation formats.

Outcomes Results

All previous areas lead to what the audience is most interested in—the results of the project described in the outcomes results section. Whether presenting the results in written or oral form, be sure to focus on this segment by making it the longest of a written report or by allotting ample time in an oral presentation. Although the outcomes step of data management takes the shortest amount of time to execute, it should encompass the largest percentage of space/time during presentation. It is essential to report the results of all aims and outcomes, whether or not they are in the desired direction or statistically significant.

The outcomes section of the analysis should be framed within the original aims and outcomes. The easiest way to report this section is in this order for each aim/outcome combination:

1. State the aim and outcome.
2. Describe the results of the outcome without adjusting for confounding.
3. Explain the results of the outcome with adjustment for confounding.

Figure 9.2 shows an example of reporting of outcomes in this format. This example summarizes the results of the example in Table 8.3 in Chapter 8.

"The first aim of this project is to improve weight management in those receiving the intervention. One outcome associated with this aim is to have 5% less patients in the intervention group with a body mass index (BMI) equal to or greater than 25 when compared to the comparison group. Figure 9.2 shows the proportion of those with a BMI equal to or greater than 25 in each group. Figure 9.2 shows that the intervention group has 86.5% (95% confidence interval [CI] = 84.3%, 88.7%) of patients with a BMI equal to or greater than 25, whereas the comparison group has 87.9% (95% CI = 85.7%, 90.2%). These results are not statistically significant ($p = .36$, using chi-square). Adjusting the results for gender using logistic regression, the intervention group is found to be less likely to have a BMI equal to or greater than 25; however, these results were not statistically significant—odds ratio (95% CI) = 0.92 (0.70, 1.21)."

Summary of Results

The summary of results highlights all the most pertinent findings in one to two paragraphs. This section is not an interpretation of results; rather it can be thought of as the "elevator speech" that summarizes the entire results. The summary is reported in a nonbiased, nonsubjective, noninterpretive, fact-based manner and

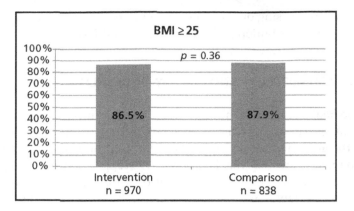

FIGURE 9.2   Reporting outcomes example.

should minimize the use of statistics because the statistics are previously reported. Following is an example of a summary of results:

"The results indicate significant improvements for the intervention group in the rates of 7 of the 13 quality measures, although only 2 of these measures demonstrate improvements for the intervention group that are significantly larger than the changes exhibited for the comparison group, LDL-C (low-density lipoprotein cholesterol) screenings for diabetics and appropriate pharmaceutical treatment of hypertension. The comparison of rates for primary care provider (PCP) visits in the intervention group does not detect a significant improvement from preintervention to postintervention, although the 2% increase for the intervention group is significantly better than the 4% decrease detected for the comparison group."

Describing Data-Related Limitations

This segment is a description of the limitations occurring at any point of the data management process that may have an impact on the ability to carry out the data analysis plan. Describing the limitations is important because it shows that the DNP understands and acknowledges that unforeseen (or suspected) circumstances may impact results, and it allows the audience to consider limitations in interpreting the results. It is meaningful to note that this section is not referring to limitations that are related to execution of the project intervention. It is also essential to mention that this section should not go into great detail to explain the reason why limitations may have occurred or to make excuses. However, when explaining the limitations it is useful to detail the impact that each limitation may have on the data management process. Some common types of data-related limitations include:

- Lack of statistical power such that the sample size is not large enough to achieve statistical significance
- Inability to collect data as planned or errors in data collection
- Ineffectiveness in executing the data management plan as designed
- Inability to match the desired data definition when using secondary data sources, resulting in the use of proxy measures (e.g., the use of zip code to infer socioeconomic status)

- Large amounts of missing data for certain measures
- Unexpected data distribution (e.g., skewed data, outliers)

IMPORTANT ASPECTS OF VISUALIZATION AND DISPLAY OF RESULTS

Presenting the final results of the translation project, it is important to use a method of display that clearly and concisely presents the important facts and immediately draws the audience's attention to those facts. If the reader takes more than 30 seconds to interpret results, that is probably too long. Choosing the appropriate format for presenting the results is the art of data management and takes some practice. Graphs and tables are the basic formats for communicating and displaying the results of the project.

Graphs

A graph is used to display quantitative information with values shown in an area with one or more axes and with values encoded as visual objects positioned in relation to the axes. The scales on the axes of the graph are used to assign values and labels to the visual objects within the graph (Few, 2004a). Graphs should be used to simply and effectively display what would be a large amount of difficult-to-understand information if described solely in text form. The best use of graphs is when conveying:

- A comparison among two or more groupings
  - For example, mean costs for the intervention and comparison groups by age categories
- Changes in values over time
  - For instance, the monthly readmission rate
- The distribution of values for a variable
  - To illustrate, the distribution of costs
- A correlation between two variables
  - For example, the relationship between age and health risk scores
- The distribution of parts to a whole
  - For instance, the proportion of total health care dollars spent inpatient versus outpatient (Conference of European Statisticians, 2009b)

A graph should "speak a thousand words" when expressing key results but should not try to convey so much information that it becomes confusing and uninterpretable. A high-quality graph captures the reader's attention; presents information clearly and accurately; does not mislead; displays the data as succinctly as possible (i.e., one graph as opposed to multiple graphs for the same information); and facilitates data comparison, highlighting trends, and differences (Conference of European Statisticians, 2009a). As part of an entire reporting of results, the use of graphs should be reserved for displaying the most important results with key impact.

Table 9.1 discusses some types and best uses of graphs that are commonly utilized when displaying the results of DNP projects.

TABLE 9.1   Common Types of Graphs and Common Uses for Reporting the Results of DNP Projects

Graph Type	Common Use for DNP Result Reporting
Point plot	Used to show specific data points. Plots can be used to display the values for one variable, for groupings of a variable, or to show the relationship between two variables. The key point is that individual data points are displayed. One example is Figure 7.13. A good use of plots is in displaying the correlation between two continuous variables (outcome variable on the y axis and independent variable on the x axis). The normal P-P plot of the observed values (independent variable) against the expected values (dependent variable) for BMI in Figure 8.7 is an example of this.
Histogram	Histograms are commonly used for describing frequency distributions or the patterns of values for interval or ratio level data. They are most commonly seen with vertical bars (although the bars can be horizontally displayed). Histograms are most often used during EDA. Figure 7.8 is an example of a histogram.
Boxplot	Boxplots are also used for describing frequency distributions. Compared to histograms, they provide more information about the distribution itself such as the median, quartiles, outliers, and extreme outliers. Boxplots are most commonly used during EDA. They can also be used during final presentation, when information about the distribution of an outcome is relevant and important for understanding the results of the project. Figure 7.9 is an example of a boxplot.
Bar graph	There are multiple displays for bar graphs, such as stacked and clustered bars. The basic use of bar graphs is to display summary information such as means and percentages for groupings or categories of another variable (e.g., when displaying the mean costs for age category groupings). A good example of a stacked bar graph is in the display of regions in the case study section of Chapter 7.
Line graph	A line graph is the most effective tool for showing trends in data over time and is ideal for showing any type of time series data. The statistical process control and run charts in Chapter 10 are all good examples.

BMI, body mass index; EDA, exploratory data analysis; P-P plot, probability-probability plot.
Source: Few (2004a) and Conference of European Statisticians (2009b).

Tables

A table organizes and displays information by arranging data that is coded in text and numbers, and in rows and columns. The primary benefit of tables is that data can be individually identified and considered (Few, 2004a). Tables are most advantageous when: (a) it is important to look up individual values; (b) it would be useful to compare individual values; (c) precise values are necessary; and (d) quantitative information to be communicated involves more than one unit of measure (Few, 2004a). Essential components of a table include:

- Title—a clear, concise, and accurate description above the table that tells the "where," "what," and "when" of the data

TABLE 9.2 Basic Table Structure

Table Title						
	Column Header	Column Header	Column Header	Column Header	Column Header	Column Header
Row Stub	Data	Data	Data	Data	Data	Data
Row Stub	Data	Data	Data	Data	Data	Data
Row Stub	Data	Data	Data	Data	Data	Data
Row Stub	Data	Data	Data	Data	Data	Data
Footnotes						
Source						

Adapted from Conference of European Statisticians (2009b).

- Column headers—descriptors at the top of each column of the table that identify the data present in each column
- Row stubs—the first column of the table, identifying the data presented in each row
- Footnotes—under the table, providing any additional information needed to understand and use the data correctly (Conference of European Statisticians, 2009b)
- Source line—under the table, appropriately references data sources

The text that is used for the title, column headers, row stubs, and footnotes is chosen carefully to perform any of the following functions: label, introduce, explain, reinforce, highlight, sequence, recommend, or inquire. These functions provide important information that relays the table's message (Few, 2004b). Table 9.2 depicts a basic table structure.

SUMMARY

This chapter describes the basic elements that need to be compiled for the reporting of DNP project data management and results along with some strategies, formats, and methods. Variation is expected in the actual communication and presentation of this information, based on the targeted audience and message.

REFERENCES

Conference of European Statisticians. (2009a). *Making data meaningful Part 1: A guide to writing stories about numbers.* New York, NY: United Nations Economic Commission for Europe.
Conference of European Statisticians. (2009b). *Making data meaningful Part 2: A guide to writing stories about numbers.* New York, NY: United Nations Economic Commission for Europe.

CONSORT Group. (n.d.). *Flow diagram: CONSORT: Transparent reporting of trials*. Retrieved September 13, 2013, from http://www.consort-statement.org/consort-statement/flow-diagram0

Few, S. (2004a). Fundamental concepts of tables and graphs. In S. Few, *Show me the numbers: Designing tables and graphs to enlighten* (pp. 38–54). Oakland, CA: Analytics Press.

Few, S. (2004b). Table design. In S. Few, *Show me the numbers: Designing tables and graphs to enlighten* (pp. 131–165). Oakland, CA: Analytics Press.

Iezzoni, L. I. (2003). *Risk adjustment for measuring healthcare outcomes*. Chicago, IL: Health Administration Press.

Ishani, A., Greer, N., Taylor, B. C., Kubes, L., Cole, P., Atwood, M., . . . Ercan-Fang, N. (2011). Effect of nurse case management compared with usual care on controlling cardiovascular risk factors in patients with diabetes. *Diabetes Care, 34*(8), 1689–1694.

Johns Hopkins Bloomberg School of Public Health. (2012). *The Johns Hopkins ACG system*. Retrieved September 21, 2013, from http://acg.jhsph.org

Moher, D., Schulz, K. F., & Altman, D. (2001). The CONSORT statement: Revised recommendations for improving the quality of reports of parallel-group randomized trials. *Annals of Internal Medicine, 134*(8), 657–662.

Schulz, K. F., Altman, D. G., & Moher, D. (2010). CONSORT 2010 statement: Updated guidelines for reporting parallel group randomised trials. *British Medical Journal, 340*, 698–702.

Sylvia, M. L., Griswold, M., Dunbar, L., Boyd, C. M., Park, M., & Boult, C. (2008). Guided care: Cost and utilization outcomes in a pilot study. *Disease Management, 11*(1), 29–36.

Welch, G., Garb, J., Zagarins, S., Lendel, I., & Gabbay, R. (2010). Nurse diabetes case management interventions and blood glucose control: Results of a meta-analysis. *Diabetes Research and Clinical Practice, 88*(1), 1–6.

CASE STUDY

CASE STUDY EXAMPLE: FINAL RESULTS

The purpose of this DNP quality improvement project is to improve the health status and the efficiency of health care resource use in older community-dwelling patients with diabetes. There are two components to this project necessitating measurement of two separate units of analysis. The first unit of analysis is older Care1 health plan community-dwelling patients 65 or older with diabetes. In this population, those in geographic region A receive the intervention; those in geographic region B do not receive the intervention and are used as a comparison group. Patients are excluded from both groups if they have a diagnosis of end-stage renal disease, are currently scheduled for an organ transplant, or are actively receiving cancer treatment.

Aims and outcomes in this population are:

Aim 1

- Older patients with diabetes to achieve and maintain appropriate control of their blood glucose levels
  - *Outcome 1a*: The intervention group has a lower mean hemoglobin A1C (HbA1C) postintervention value when matched against the comparison group. Based on evidence from a pilot study at this intervention site and considering corroboration from the literature, the expected difference in mean HbA1C levels is approximately 0.9 (Ishani et al., 2011; Welch, Garb, Zagarins, Lendel, & Gabbay, 2010).
  - *Outcome 1b*: The intervention group has a larger mean lowering of HbA1C values from preintervention to postintervention when contrasted with the comparison group. Based on clinical experience, the expected difference in mean lowering between both groups is approximately 25%.

Aim 2

- Older patients with diabetes to experience efficient use of health care services
  - *Outcome 2a*: The intervention group has lower mean inpatient hospitalizations postintervention compared to the comparison group. Based on available evidence and clinical experience, the expected difference in means is at least .20 admissions per year (Sylvia et al., 2008).
  - *Outcome 2b*: The intervention group has a lower percentage of patients with any hospitalization in the postperiod when matched against the comparison group. Based on limited available evidence and clinical experience, the difference in percentages is expected to be approximately 50%.
  - *Outcome 2c*: The intervention group has a larger mean lowering of inpatient admissions from preintervention to postintervention when equated with the comparison group. Based on clinical experience, the difference in mean lowering between both groups is at least 50%.

In order to determine the sample size necessary for this project, the following aims and outcomes are used:

Aim 1: Outcome 1a

The inputs and output for this power analysis are:

Alpha: equals 0.05
Power: equals 0.80
Standard deviation or sigma: equals 1.5
Difference in means: equals 0.9
Calculated sample size: equals 45

Aim 2: Outcome 2a

The inputs and output for this power analysis are:

Alpha: equals 0.05
Power: equals 0.80
Standard deviation or sigma: equals 0.8
Difference in means: equals 0.2
Calculated sample size: equals 255

In summary, detecting a statistically significant difference in the HbA1C mean (aim 1, outcome 1a) requires a sample size of 45 in each group. In order to detect a statistically significant difference in mean admissions (aim 2, outcome 2a), a sample size of 255 is needed in each group. The constraints of this project are such that the maximum expected amount of patients in each group is no greater than 200. This means that the project sample size is high enough to detect a statistically significant difference in the mean HbA1C between groups but likely not powered to detect a statistically significant difference in the mean number of admissions between groups.

The second unit of analysis is admissions for all community-dwelling patients with diabetes who are enrolled in a Care1 health plan for 1 full year following a statewide initiative to reduce readmission rates. Admissions to a skilled nursing facility are excluded. A total of 3,500 admissions are estimated.

Aims and outcomes in this population are:

Aim 3

- All Care1 health plan older patients with diabetes to experience efficient use of health care services
  - *Outcome 3a*: Care1 health plan patients with diabetes have less than a 15% rate of 30-day readmissions in the postperiod, based on published local benchmark data.

This outcome is descriptive and therefore no power analysis is performed.

Flow of Patients

For the intervention group and the comparison group each, 220 patients are identified within the community-dwelling patient population with diabetes. Within the intervention group, 10 of the 220 do not meet the inclusion/exclusion criteria and 2 are later removed due to disenrollment from the health plan—leaving a final total of 208. Of those originally identified for the comparison group, 32 do not meet the inclusion/exclusion criteria and 4 disenrolled from the health plan—leaving a final total of 184.

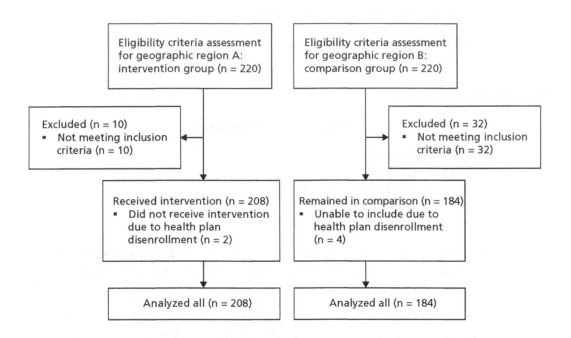

An analysis of Care1 health plan's admission data reveals 4,152 admissions meeting the criteria for analysis. During the process of data cleansing, 44 duplicate admissions are removed—leaving a final total number of 4,108 admissions.

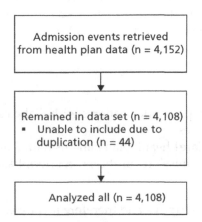

Data Collection

Secondary data sources are used for both data sets and all variables within those data sets. Care1 health plan receives enrollment information from patients enrolling in the health plan; billing information from health care providers and facilities that provide health care services to their health plan membership; pharmacy information from pharmacies providing medications for patients; and laboratory and radiology results from companies providing those services. Enrollment data contain patient name, address, enrollment and disenrollment dates, reason for eligibility, and specific benefit-package information. Billing data for patient health care services contain detailed facts about the: diagnosis of the patient, service provided, facility where the service is given, provider(s) involved in delivering the services, time and date of the service, and cost of the service. Pharmacy data are also billing data but specifically for outpatient pharmacy products. These data contain information about the name, type, class, dosage, route of administration, amount, and brand of the drug provided to the patient. Laboratory and radiology data give facts about the type of test done and the results of that test. Care1 health plan combines all of this information into a queryable database.

The Adjusted Clinical Groups® (ACG) system is a person-focused method of categorizing patients' constellations of illnesses into a single group or ACG, providing a measure of the effect of illness burden. Morbidity burden is classified using complex electronic algorithms based on the duration, severity, diagnostic certainty, etiology, and specialty care needs of an individual as well as age and gender (Johns Hopkins Bloomberg School of Public Health, 2012). The risk adjustment score used in this project is derived using the ACG methodology. Care1 health plan runs the ACG software and keeps a historical record of output of patient ACG variables.

Care1 health plan provides databases to evaluate this project, the success of the aims of the intervention for the older community-dwelling population, and for the admission events falling within the statewide initiative to reduce inpatient readmission rates. The data set for the senior community-dwelling population is provided in the final analysis data set structure outlined in the evaluation plan. The data set for the readmissions evaluation is presented in a format that requires some data manipulation to create a final analysis data set.

Data Governance

This project and its evaluation are approved by the Care1 health plan institutional review board (IRB), with an obtained waiver of consent. A limited data set—defined by the Health Insurance Portability and Accountability Act (HIPAA) as one that has all direct identifiers removed—is used for the analysis. The data for this project are maintained and analyzed on Care1 health plan servers, with no data being taken out of the Care1 health plan secure data environment.

Data Cleansing and Manipulation

The data set for the older community-dwelling population is provided in the final analysis data set structure outlined in the evaluation plan. However the final outcome variables that measure the difference in pre/post-admissions, difference in pre-/post-HbA1C, and occurrence of an admission in the postperiod are calculated from provided data.

The data set for the readmissions evaluation requires more manipulation and cleansing. First, the required date fields are created from the separated year, month, and date fields. Next, 44 duplicate admissions are identified and removed from the data set. These removed admissions are actually determined to be a subset of one continuous admission—often the result of a transfer between facilities or units within one facility. A variable is then created to determine the number of days between any one admission and the subsequent admission. This new variable is used to determine whether each admission in the data set is actually a readmission. A readmission is defined as any admission occurring less than 30 days following a previous admission for the same patient.

Results of Data Analysis for Community-Dwelling Older Patients With Diabetes

The following table shows the differences in means and proportions for the demographic characteristics, morbidity level, and certain illness prevalence between the intervention group and the comparison group. The intervention group has a higher percentage of patients in the high-risk and very-high-risk morbidity category compared to the comparison group (74.0% vs. 64.7%, $p < .05$). The prevalence of comorbidities is similar between both groups—except for cancer, where the intervention group has a rate of 9.1% and the comparison group has a rate of 17.4% ($p < .05$), and diabetic retinopathy, where the intervention group has a rate of 12.5% and the comparison group has a rate of 6.5%.

Demographic and Descriptive Characteristics of the Older Community-Dwelling Population

Characteristic	Intervention	Comparison
Number in group	208	184
Age mean (range)*	74.4 (65–100)	74.9 (65–96)
% Women	44.0%	38.9%
Race		
% White	43.3%	46.2%
% African American/Black	51.9%	52.7%
% Hispanic	4.8%	1.1%
Morbidity level**		
% Low risk	0.5%	2.2%
% Moderate risk	25.5%	33.2%
% High risk	39.4%	43.5%
% Very high risk	34.6%	21.2%

(continued)

Demographic and Descriptive Characteristics of the Older Community-Dwelling Population (*continued*)

Characteristic	Intervention	Comparison
% AMI	3.4%	3.8%
% Anxiety/neurosis	5.8%	10.3%
% Asthma	2.9%	3.3%
% Blindness	1.0%	0.5%
% Cancer*	**9.1%**	**17.4%**
% Cardiac arrest	1.0%	1.1%
% Cardiomyopathy	2.4%	1.1%
% Cerebrovascular disease	13.0%	14.7%
% Chronic liver disease	0.5%	0.5%
% Chronic pancreatitis	1.0%	0.5%
% Chronic renal failure	10.1%	9.2%
% Chronic skin ulcer	3.4%	2.2%
% Congestive heart failure	11.1%	10.9%
% Degenerative joint disease	38.0%	31.0%
% Dementia/delirium	5.8%	6.0%
% Depression	8.2%	10.9%
% Diabetic retinopathy*	**12.5%**	**6.5%**
% Disorder of lipoid metabolism	75.0%	75.0%
% Emphysema/chronic bronchitis/COPD	6.7%	11.4%
% Generalized atherosclerosis	27.9%	23.4%
% Glaucoma	24.5%	29.3%
% Hypertension	79.3%	85.3%
% Ischemic heart disease	25.0%	28.8%
% Obesity	21.6%	15.2%
% Ophthalmic signs/symptoms	2.4%	1.1%
% Parkinson's disease	1.4%	1.6%
% Peripheral neuropathy	13.5%	15.2%
% Tobacco use	4.3%	4.3%
% Transplant	0.5%	0.5%

***Bold values** represent $p < .05$ using t-test for continuous variables and chi-square for categorical variable.

**Assumptions for chi-square are not met when morbidity burden is broken down into these reported categories. The chi-square test is significant when dichotomizing variable and assumptions are met.

AMI, acute myocardial infarction; COPD, chronic obstructive pulmonary disease.

Exploratory data analysis reveals that for two of the outcome measures—"mean HbA1C in the postperiod" and "mean number of admissions in the postperiod"—the distributions do not meet the assumptions necessary for parametric statistical testing. Hence, these measures are tested using nonparametric methods.

Thoughtful review of the exploratory analysis for this population indicates that morbidity level is a confounder of the relationship between the intervention and admissions-related outcomes when dichotomized into two categories: one indicative of "high risk" and "very high risk" and the second indicative of "moderate risk" and "low risk." Dichotomization is necessary due to the skewed distribution of morbidity level in each group. The following table shows the difference between those with high and low morbidity for the project outcomes in which parametric statistical testing is performed.

The Effect of Morbidity Burden on Outcomes

Morbidity Group	Difference in Pre-/ Post-HbA1C, p = .139	Difference in Pre/Post-Admissions, p = .001	Presence of an Admission in the Postperiod, p = .000
High morbidity	Mean (SD), (95% CI) 0.41 (1.94), (0.18–0.64)	Mean (SD), (95% CI) 0.07 (1.32), (-0.08–0.23)	% High morbidity, (95% CI) 36.0%, (31.0%–42.0%)
Low morbidity	Mean (SD), (95% CI) 0.09 (1.93), (-0.26 – 0.44)	Mean (SD), (95% CI) -0.29 (0.86), (-0.45 – [-0.14])	% Low morbidity, (95% CI) 5.0%, (1.0%–9.0%)

CI, confidence interval; HbA1C, hemoglobin A1C; SD, standard deviation.

Each outcome is tested without any adjustment for confounding and reveals the following results:

Unadjusted Results of Outcomes for Community-Dwelling Seniors With Diabetes Quality Improvement Project

Outcome	Intervention	Comparison	Statistical Test and Result
HbA1C in the postperiod, mean per patient (SD), (95% CI), median	7.86 (1.54), (7.69, 8.03), 7.70	8.30 (1.41), (8.10, 8.50), 7.70	Mann-Whitney U test p = .009
Pre-/post-HbA1C difference, mean per patient (SD), (95% CI)	-0.09 (1.85), (-0.34, 0.17)	0.76 (1.95), (0.47, 1.04)	Independent t-test p < .001
No. of admissions in the postperiod, mean per patient (SD), (95% CI), median	0.29 (0.68), (0.20, 0.38), 0.00	0.55 (0.91), (0.42, 0.69), 0.00	Mann-Whitney U test p = .001
Difference in no. of pre/ post-admissions, mean per patient (SD), (95% CI)	-0.14 (0.83), (-0.26, 0.03)	0.08 (1.53), (-0.14, 0.30)	Independent t-test p = .075
Indicator of an admission in the postperiod, %, (95% CI)	19.7% (0.83), (14.3%, 25.2%)	34.8% (27.8%, 44.7%)	Chi-square test p = .001

CI, confidence interval; HbA1C, hemoglobin A1C; SD, standard deviation.

The intervention group has a lower mean HbA1C per patient in the postperiod compared to the comparison group (7.86 vs. 8.30). The differences in HbA1C are statistically significant using the Mann-Whitney U nonparametric rank test ($p = .009$). The intervention group has a mean decrease of 0.09 in the pre-/post-HbA1C value per patient, whereas the comparison group has a mean increase of 0.76 ($p < .001$).

The intervention group has a lower mean number of admissions per patient in the postperiod compared to the comparison group (0.29 vs. 0.55). The differences in number of admissions per patient are statistically significant using the Mann-Whitney U nonparametric rank test ($p = .001$). The intervention group has a mean decrease of 0.14 pre/post-admissions per patient, although the comparison group has a mean increase of 0.08; however, these results are not statistically significant ($p = .075$). Within the intervention group, 19.7% of patients have an admission; 34.8% of those in the comparison group have an admission. These results are significant ($p = .001$).

Each outcome meeting the requirements of parametric statistical testing is then tested using regression analysis adjusting for the confounding effect of morbidity level. Following are the obtained results:

Impact of the Intervention on Outcomes Adjusted for Patient Morbidity Level*

Outcome	Mean or Odds Ratio	95% Confidence Interval	p Value	Model Statistic
Change in mean pre-/ post-HbA1C value per patient	-0.88	(-1.26, -0.51)	($p < .001$)	$R^2 = 5.7\%$
Change in mean no. of pre/post-admissions per patient	-0.26	(-0.50, -0.02)	($p = .031$)	$R^2 = 3.1\%$
Odds of an admission in the postperiod	0.36	(0.21, -0.57)	($p < .001$)	Hosmer-Lemeshow $p = .365$

*Linear regression is used for continuous outcomes and logistic regression for dichotomous outcomes. HbA1C, hemoglobin A1C; R^2, coefficient of determination.

Adjusted for morbidity level, the change in HbA1C values is on average 0.88 points lower per patient for those in the intervention group versus the comparison group ($p < .001$). The difference in number of admissions is on average 0.26 lower per patient for those in the intervention group versus the comparison group adjusted for morbidity level ($p = .031$). The odds of having an admission are 0.36 times (or 64% less) for those in the intervention group versus the comparison group adjusted for morbidity level ($p < .001$).

Results of Data Analysis for Admissions of Community-Dwelling Patients With Diabetes in Care1 Health Plan

There are a total of 4,108 admissions in the data set for the community-dwelling patients with diabetes who are enrolled in Care1 health plan for 1 full year following the implementation of the readmissions prevention initiative. Of these 4,108 admissions, 17.6% ($n = 722$) are readmissions. Descriptive information shows that:

- Patients
  - A total of 2,470 patients account for the 4,108 total admissions.
  - Of the total 2,470 patients, 13% (*n* = 309) account for the 722 readmissions, leaving 87% of the total patients with no readmission.
- Age
  - The distribution of age is right skewed for all admissions and readmissions. The median age for admissions and readmissions is the same, with the distribution of age for overall admissions having many older outliers than the distribution for readmissions.

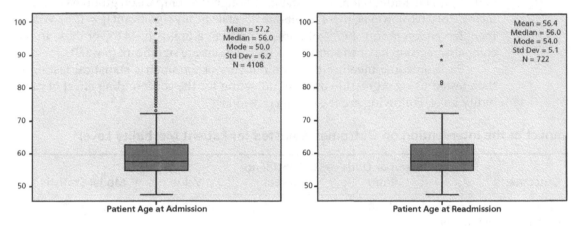

- Gender
  - Women—55.3% of all admissions
  - Women—43.4% of all readmissions
- Diagnosis-related group (DRG) classifications
  - A wide variety of DRGs account for admissions and readmissions, with the highest-frequency DRG (chronic obstructive pulmonary disease [COPD]) associated with only 6.4% of overall admissions. Only the top 15 frequent DRGs are shown in the next table. A total of 237 DRGs are present in all of the admissions and a total of 156 DRGs are present in the readmissions.

Total Admissions N = 4,108			Readmissions N = 722		
DRG	Frequency	Percent	DRG	Frequency	Percent
Chronic obstructive pulmonary disease	264	6.4	Chronic obstructive pulmonary disease	53	7.3
Heart failure	156	3.8	Heart failure	41	5.7
Knee joint replacement	137	3.3	Pulmonary edema & respiratory failure	25	3.5
Septicemia & disseminated infections	104	2.5	Septicemia & disseminated infections	25	3.5
Other pneumonia	102	2.5	Disorders of pancreas except malignancy	19	2.6
Cellulitis & other bacterial skin infections	98	2.4	Electrolyte disorders except hypovolemia related	17	2.4

Total Admissions N = 4,108			Readmissions N = 722		
DRG	Frequency	Percent	DRG	Frequency	Percent
Disorders of pancreas except malignancy	83	2.0	Renal failure	17	2.4
Renal failure	81	2.0	Cellulitis & other bacterial skin infections	15	2.1
Hip joint replacement	77	1.9	Other pneumonia	15	2.1
Pulmonary edema & respiratory failure	67	1.6	Diabetes	14	1.9
CVA & precerebral occlusion w infarct	66	1.6	Peptic ulcer & gastritis	14	1.9
Cardiac arrhythmia & conduction disorders	63	1.5	Hepatic coma & other major acute liver disorders	13	1.8
Diabetes	62	1.5	HIV w major HIV related conditions	13	1.8
Electrolyte disorders except hypovolemia related	56	1.4	HIV w multiple major HIV related conditions	13	1.8
Seizure	56	1.4	Peripheral & other vascular disorders	13	1.8

- Bed type
  - The majority of admissions and readmissions occur within two bed types (medical and intensive care).

Bed Type	All Admissions (%)	Readmissions (%)
Medical	81.5	79.5
Intensive care unit	16.1	18.0
Acute rehab	1.2	1.5
Psychiatric	0.7	0.6
Other	0.3	0.4
Obstetrics	0.2	0.0
Subacute	0.1	0.0

- Readmissions
  - Of the overall 4,108 admissions, 722 are readmissions—a rate of 17.6%.

Summary of Results

The results of the intervention providing intensive care management services to older community-dwelling patients with diabetes are positive. The intervention group overall has a lower mean HbA1C per patient following the intervention and a lowering of the HbA1C from the start to the end of the intervention versus the comparison group. Additionally, those receiving the intervention have fewer admissions in the postperiod, a lowering of the number of admissions, and a lower percentage of patients with an admission in the postperiod. Adjusting for morbidity burden—which was higher in the intervention group—these results are consistent and statistically significant; nevertheless, model statistics show that much of the variability in these outcomes is still unaccounted for.

The statewide initiative to reduce readmissions for community-dwelling senior adults with diabetes does not meet the desired benchmark of a 15% or lower readmission rate. Descriptive information about readmissions shows that a small percentage of the entirety of patients with an admission accounts for the readmissions. In a wide variety of assigned diagnostic categories for admissions and readmissions, COPD and heart failure account for the highest percentages.

Data Limitations

This evaluation is powered to find anticipated differences in mean HbA1C levels per patient but not anticipated differences in mean admissions per patient. As it turns out, the skewed distributions of the HbA1C values and number of admissions in the postperiod do not allow for means testing of these measures. However, the realized unadjusted differences in each measure are larger than expected, leading to statistically significant differences in all of the unadjusted measures except for the difference in the number of pre/post-admissions.

Known errors in data acquisition and missing data elements are minimal. A small percentage of duplicate hospitalizations have been removed from the readmissions data. It is important to note that the administrative claims data used for this analysis is a subset of data created for billing and payment for services and not for evaluation purposes. As such, data for each patient can change over time if a claim is appealed or reversed, a correction is made to the information on a claim, or the timing for claims submission (typically within 3 months of receiving the service) is longer than expected. Administrative claims data also suffer from under/overcoding, inaccurate coding, diagnoses lacking in clinical scope and meaningfulness, and errors in and lack of submission (Iezzoni, 2003). The morbidity level variable developed within the ACG system depends on *ICD-9-CM* (*International Classification of Diseases, Ninth Revision, Clinical Modification*) diagnoses in administrative claims data and may suffer from the same limitations.

The skewed distributions for HbA1C and admissions in the postperiod limit the ability to use means testing for these measures. It is possible that more sophisticated statistical models can be developed to handle the complex distributions for these outcomes.

CHAPTER 10

Ongoing Monitoring

MELISSA SHERRY

Data management is not a linear process. Instead, it should be thought of as an ongoing feedback loop where data gathered, analyzed, and evaluated are used to continuously inform decisions and improve processes. As processes are modified, deleted, or continued to achieve the desired outcome, data must continue to be gathered and monitored to understand ongoing effects of the intervention and make decisions to further ensure that the best possible outcomes are achieved. Many tools, including statistical process control (SPC) charts, run charts, and benchmarks, can be used by the Doctor of Nursing Practice (DNP) student to understand intervention techniques and outcomes. These tools should be employed as part of a broader and ongoing continuous quality improvement (CQI) effort to ensure that gaps in the intervention are responded to and weak areas are addressed throughout the life of the intervention.

LEARNING OBJECTIVES

After reading this chapter, the DNP should be able to:

- Understand the need and use for ongoing monitoring
- Comprehend and interpret SPC methods for ongoing data monitoring
- Choose appropriate benchmarks and utilize them to understand progress and goals of program data
- Create a CQI process to troubleshoot problems and help improve processes to achieve desired outcomes

THE NEED FOR ONGOING MONITORING

For the purposes of this chapter, ongoing monitoring is the process by which a team collects, analyzes, and utilizes data on processes and preliminary outcomes of an intervention in order to manage, understand, and improve an intervention. Ongoing monitoring of program outcomes is a continuous process that should occur as long as any intervention is in place, after the initial understanding of data

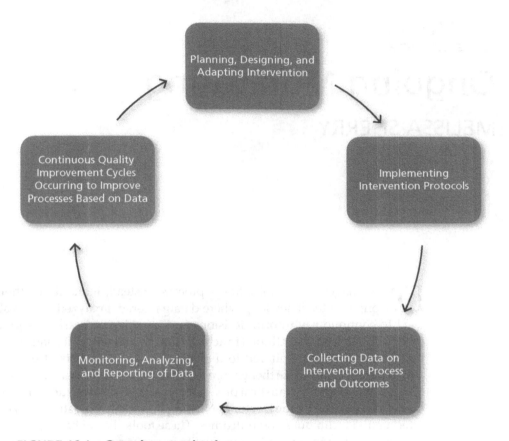

FIGURE 10.1   Ongoing monitoring.

has been accomplished (in the early evaluative phase of evidence translation) and the decision has been made to continue the project. Once an intervention has been implemented and evaluated, results are used to change or modify protocols as needed to improve the program and collect more data. This process demonstrates how examination of outcomes is a circular and not a linear process; with new changes in place, the evaluation phase evolves into a circular process of ongoing monitoring. Figure 10.1 shows how each step informs the next in a circular process.

GOALS OF ONGOING MONITORING

Ongoing monitoring is important for several reasons. First, before interpreting results of any program, one must ensure the procedures are running according to protocol in order to correctly attribute outcomes to the program. This continuous monitoring should be implemented with a clear understanding of the program's goals. For example, in a patient safety initiative related to hospital-acquired infections, a goal would be to see the number of infections drop to a certain level. (This level may be set through establishing a percentage-reduction desired based on current levels or through comparison with a benchmark to establish an appropriate goal.) Benchmarking is covered in detail in a later section of this chapter.

During ongoing monitoring, the intervention team would define, select, and monitor process measures to ensure that the intervention for reducing infections is being carried out in a consistent manner according to intervention protocols. For instance, if the process involves the use of checklists by surgeons, one would need to make sure that use of checklists is standardized and consistent across each surgeon participating in the intervention group. Only then would it be possible to determine whether program outcomes are related to that process.

In addition to understanding whether or not processes are being performed in the way they are designed, another important reason for ongoing monitoring is that various stakeholders require regular information to manage and make decisions regarding the intervention. For any intervention delivered in a health care setting, there are many stakeholders, and each one has different priorities and information needs. These stakeholders include payers, managers, providers, accreditation boards, community partners, policymakers, and other health care professionals who may require regular information throughout the life of the project, in addition to the data gathered on outcomes or results from an evaluation done at later points in the intervention. Stakeholders need timely and meaningful data about the process and outcomes of a program on a regular basis to inform decisions such as whether or not to expand a program, whether or not to change or discontinue certain aspects of a program, or to inform quality improvement (QI) processes. This is discussed later in this chapter.

CHALLENGES IN ONGOING MONITORING

Designing ongoing monitoring plans can be quite a challenge, given these various stakeholder interests. One of the principal challenges in monitoring a new program is generating actionable data related to whether or not the program is having the intended effects on the population of interest. Although evaluations use rigorous methods to determine if a program is having the desired effects, these are often time-consuming. An evaluation may require many months of data; thus, it is often not done until about 6 months to 1 year after full implementation. Whereas evaluations are extremely important to understanding interventions, they may not be timely enough for stakeholders who require information to make decisions along the way.

Ongoing monitoring data should provide information to support the needs of different stakeholders. For managers and staff of the program, it is essential to know whether or not the program is being implemented according to protocol, and whether process goals such as completion of a certain number of assessments per month are being achieved. Fidelity to protocols can mean the difference between an intervention's success and failure; hence, implementation measures must be continuously produced and examined in order to ensure the intervention is being delivered as intended.

To illustrate, if an intervention involves case managers working with pregnant women to reduce preterm birthrates, monitoring of process measures such as contacts between the pregnant women and case managers, rates of prenatal care visits among the pregnant women, and appropriate use of medication therapy provides information on how well intervention processes are working to aid in interpreting key health outcomes of the program. In other words, if process

TABLE 10.1 Example of a Dashboard With Select Process and Outcome Metrics

	2013						2014					
	QTR 1			QTR 2			QTR 3			QTR 4		
	Jul	Aug	Sep	Oct	Nov	Dec	Jan	Feb	Mar	Apr	May	Jun
Process Metrics												
Identified as eligible	15	75	123	245	323	435	533	567	675	732	845	912
Outreached by case manager	1	13	45	54	68	133	198	255	268	343	492	587
Opened in intervention	0	12	34	46	55	67	96	104	136	165	171	203
Education module completed by enrollee	0	1	13	32	49	58	88	99	120	143	156	167
Outcome Metrics												
Admission rate per 1,000	232	201	176	185	211	193	232	224	198	187	199	212
Total cost of care per patient per month	$5,462	$5,233	$5,102	$4,987	$4,954	$4,766	$4,682	$4,978	$4,877	$4,454	$4,766	$4,677
Diabetic admission rate per 1,000	112	97	86	103	88	93	114	99	80	83	92	90
Emergency department visit rate per 1,000	243	235	254	233	265	276	254	243	265	238	240	246

measures are not monitored by those managing the intervention, the team cannot assume that the intervention is being delivered as designed and cannot attribute observed outcomes to the intervention.

The choice and method of data presentation for ongoing monitoring purposes should also be done according to the needs of the audience. Various stakeholders have different levels of statistical knowledge and background, and the way data are presented to stakeholders should ideally vary based on the type of information and level of necessary detail. For example, an analytical audience may appreciate dashboards of information with confidence intervals (CIs), *t*-tests, or chi-square tests included to help them understand significance in data fluctuation. An audience with less of a statistical background may be overwhelmed by these types of data and instead prefer graphs that display more easily interpreted trends. Control charts, described later in this chapter, are also a good tool for displaying data in an easily interpretable manner. These decisions should be made based on each stakeholder's requirements.

Program managers likely want detailed information on the process measures and outcome measures of the program in order to make sure the program is running as it should. They probably prefer data on a weekly or biweekly basis in the form of dashboards, graphs, or both. For examples of some formats for presenting monitoring of data, see Table 10.1 and Figure 10.2. The dashboard in Table 10.1, which tracks monthly process and outcome measures over 1 year of intervention, is an example of the type of information needed by managers. The graph in Figure 10.2 may be useful for managers, as well. This chart can also be presented to less involved stakeholders because it shows one outcome of an intervention tracked over 1 year in a quickly interpretable manner.

Unlike program managers, less involved stakeholders, such as a hospital administrator who has approved the intervention but is not part of the day-to-day operation, may want monthly or quarterly summary information presented in a succinct and easily interpretable manner: perhaps bulleted summary points

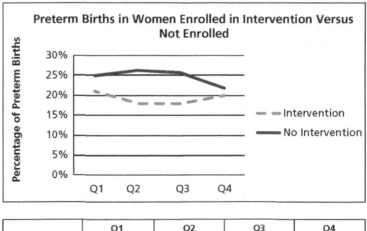

	Q1	Q2	Q3	Q4
Intervention	0.21	0.18	0.18	0.2
No intervention	0.25	0.26	0.26	0.22

FIGURE 10.2   Example of a single graph for an outcome measure.

under graphs showing only the main outcomes of the program. Higher-level stakeholders often want to stay informed of the progress of the program without getting bogged down by daily details and processes. Payers or insurers may want report-card–type data for accountability purposes. It is important to keep in mind that if an intervention is funded by a grant or outside source, these payers often have their own criteria for what should be reported for ongoing monitoring purposes and how it should be presented.

RUN CHARTS AND SPC

One of the biggest challenges in understanding tables, graphs, or other methods of displaying data on the intervention processes and outcomes over time is in determining which changes seen in the data are meaningful and which are due to normal fluctuations in processes. (Note: In this chapter, "outcomes" are considered to be clinical or utilization indicators that serve as measures for monitoring the success of processes. An example of a process is completion of a nurse intervention such as the administration of a self-management education module; and an example of an outcome measure related to that process would be better control of diabetes as determined by hemoglobin A1C [HbA1C] control measurement or reduction in unplanned utilization due to diabetes complications over time.)

Defining Variation

Natural variation in any process or outcome is variation that occurs normally, due to individual differences, social and environmental factors (e.g., seasonality), and other factors inherent in the process being measured. Natural variation makes it difficult to use t-tests or chi-square tests alone to understand changes between data points because simply comparing two data points in time does not offer a clear understanding of the natural variation basic to the process or outcome being measured. Therefore, use of these statistical tests may produce results that indicate a significant change where there is only normal fluctuation. Natural variation must be taken into consideration when interpreting data trends (Carey, 2003).

Special cause variation, on the other hand, is a type of variation that occurs from causes outside of those naturally taking place in a process. Special cause variation happens when there is a significant change in the measure—signaling that there has been a crucial change in the process that the measure represents. Whether that change is positive or negative depends on circumstances, but special cause variation can usually be assigned to specific or several factors (Carey, 2003). Determining what type of variation is occurring during ongoing monitoring of an intervention is the key to understanding whether an intervention is having the intended effects on the measures being monitored (Carey, 2003).

Run Charts

The most basic way to grasp common cause and special cause variation in data is to use a run chart, which was developed by Walter Shewhart in the 1920s as a way to assist managers at Bell Telephone Laboratories in understanding variation

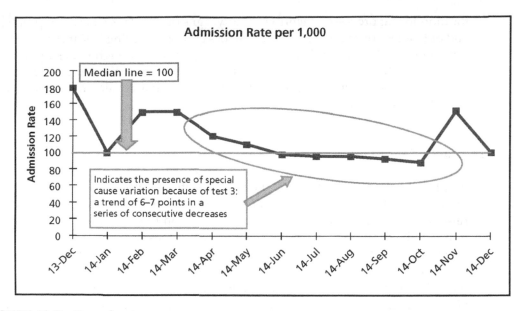

FIGURE 10.3   Run chart.

in their processes (Carey, 2003). The run chart later evolved into the SPC chart discussed in the next section (Carey, 2003). The run chart is used to plot data points of a process over time and displays each point chronologically, with a median line delineated on the graph. A "run" is defined as one or more consecutive points that are on the same side of the median line (Carey, 2003). This means that each time a point switches to the other side of the median line, it becomes a new run, or the first point in a series of points that make up a run. Using a run chart to test for special cause variation usually centers around three main tests for significance in the patterns of data points (Carey, 2003):

1. Too much or too little variability, signified by too many or too few runs
2. A shift in the process, signified by a run containing too many data points
3. The presence of a trend, defined by at least 6 to 7 points in a series of consecutive increases or decreases

Each of these tests indicates that something meaningful has occurred within the process and that the trend should be examined carefully. See Figure 10.3 for an example of a run chart with annotation to describe changes in trend.

SPC Charts

Walter Shewhart also developed another methodology for interpreting whether special cause variation is occurring in processes: SPC (Carey, 2003). SPC is a more sensitive and powerful way of displaying data over time that involves taking various methods for monitoring processes and combining them to determine whether changes seen in the data over time are statistically significantly different from normal variation (indicative of special cause variation). The SPC charts are useful for monitoring processes, identifying early signs of correlation between processes and outcomes, identifying differences across groups, or aiding in self-management interventions (Marsteller, Huizinga, & Cooper, 2013). Although not as rigorous as a full evaluation, SPC offers a shorter-term method for monitoring programs to determine whether meaningful changes are taking place following implementation of an intervention.

Benefits and Limitations of SPC

Employing SPC methods avoids the lack of statistical power issues often resulting from small sample sizes, meaning these charts are also useful for measuring rare events and for providing early information on the outcomes of an intervention. Unlike most other statistical methods, SPC does not require a large sample size for each data point to understand significance in observed changes. Instead, SPC requires multiple chronological data points, and combines statistical methods with time sensitivity to understand the significance of changes chronologically (Thor et al., 2007). This means that one can use small sample sizes—even changes to a single person's blood pressure over a period of time, for example—if there are enough points in time to meet the 20-point to 24-point minimum needed to establish common variation (Carey, 2003).

SPC charts simplify interpretation of data, making such charts ideal for displaying data for all types of audiences. It is important to realize, however, that SPC charts have the following limitations; they require many data points over time, need smart application to be used effectively, and involve some degree of autocorrelation (Benneyan, Lloyd, & Plsek, 2003; Marsteller et al., 2013).

SPC charts use principals of statistics to create measures of variation that allow distinguishing between common cause variation and special cause variation. To illustrate, implementation of a program, a change in a process, or external events such as a flu outbreak can all be causes of special cause variation. Looking for evidence that an intervention is having intended effects, one either wants to see special cause variation—as in the case of an intervention to reduce readmissions, where a change in readmission rates is desired—or wishes to see no signs of special cause variation—as in the case of an example of a patient safety initiative aimed at maintaining a minimum number of hospital-acquired infections.

Creating and Interpreting SPC Charts

To plot SPC charts, one must plot the quantitative value on the y axis and the time interval on the x axis, with means and standard deviations calculated for the quantitative values to create upper control limits (UCLs) and lower control limits (LCLs). The simplest way to create such charts is to use SPC software because it will calculate UCLs and LCLs for the data based on the chart type selected. There are many types of SPC charts, including the P, U, C, I, X-bar, and S charts, each of which should be chosen carefully depending on the type of data available for the measure of interest (Carey, 2003). Many types of data can be used, including ordinal, interval, and ratio data, but each of these requires that a different type of chart be used to detect special cause variation.

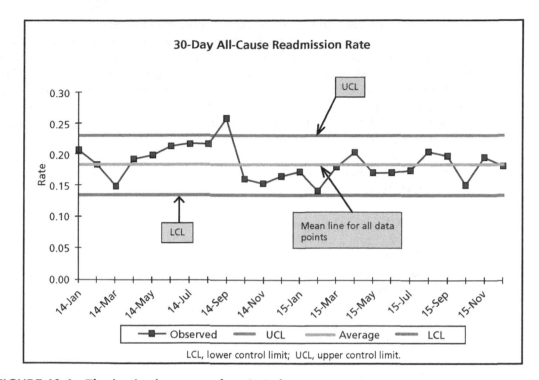

FIGURE 10.4   The basic elements of an SPC chart.

Although each chart type calculates the UCL and LCL differently, a common rule in SPC is that UCLs and LCLs represent three standard deviations above and below the mean. Refer to more comprehensive sources such as Raymond Carey's textbook *Improving Healthcare with Control Charts: Basic and Advanced SPC Methods and Case Studies* (2003) for more information on various types of control charts, how to choose the appropriate type of chart, and how to create and interpret control charts. Figure 10.4 provides a basic overview of features of a control chart.

Before creating SPC charts, one must understand the processes of interest and the measures for those processes that would provide the most useful information for understanding the intervention. For example, in an intervention aimed at reducing patient falls through provision of self-management education, one can choose to monitor the process measure of patients per month receiving self-management education and the outcome measure of the proportion of patient falls occurring among those who have received self-management education.

One measure of interest is typically chosen to display on each SPC chart (although one can choose to monitor several simultaneous processes on the same chart). It is important to choose measures for which data over time are available. Most control charts need between 20 and 35 data points in time in order to avoid Type I and Type II errors (Carey, 2003). Each data point represents data on a subgroup that can be made up of only one individual or many individuals; SPC just requires that measures are obtained over 20 points to 35 points in time. With less than 20 data points, special causes may be missed; however, with more than 35 data points, there may be multiple false–positive special causes identified (Carey, 2003). Each data point on the x axis can be represented by weeks, months, quarters, or other time intervals, although using smaller time intervals like days may lead to autocorrelation issues. This occurs when subgroups are not independent and may affect each other over time, thus increasing the number of Type I errors. Autocorrelation decreases as the time between data sampling is increased (Carey, 2003). One should consider that a number of these data points can be historical data points gathered prior to an intervention, and ideally should be, if the goal is to see a significant shift in the data points that indicates special cause variation after implementation of an intervention.

Once control charts are plotted, there is typically a set of tests to determine significance. The following tests are usually employed to evaluate for significance on SPC charts (Benneyan et al., 2003):

- Outside the UCLs or LCLs—1 point
- More than 2 sigma from the mean on the same side of the center line—2 of 3 successive points
- More than 1 sigma from the mean on the same side of the center line—4 out of 5 successive points
- On the same side of the center line—8 successive points
- Increasing or decreasing (a trend)—6 successive points
- Obvious cyclical behavior

See Figure 10.5 for an example of a trend demonstrating several examples of the tests for significance.

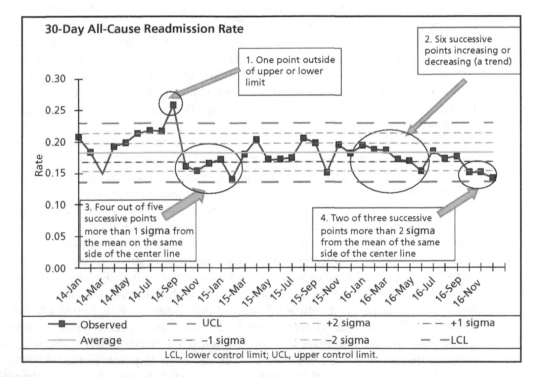

FIGURE 10.5   Tests for significance on an SPC chart.

Understanding Run Charts and SPC Charts

When one applies the tests for significance on either run charts or SPC charts and begins to see changes in variation that may indicate special cause, the next step is to understand the causes of such variation. It may be helpful to track significant events throughout the life of the intervention on the same chart as the plotted data, such as in Figure 10.6, showing an SPC chart with key events noted along the x axis in the chronological order in which they occurred. Adding timelines of when an intervention began, when a certain portion of an intervention was rolled out, or when other meaningful events occurred helps the team interpret changes seen in the data over time. If there is indication of special cause variation after an intervention began or after a change to the intervention when no other cause of the change is identified, one can attribute the special cause variation, with some confidence, to the intervention or change in intervention.

If presence of special cause variation is not something desirable, the team can strategize on ways to change the processes to avoid special cause variation in the data. For example, if an intervention has previously successfully lowered surgical infection rates to a minimum level, ongoing monitoring using SPC would ideally show that infection rates remain low with no special causes in the data that would indicate presence of significantly higher rates of infection. SPC charts should be used throughout the life of an intervention to understand the processes and begin to interpret the outcomes over time.

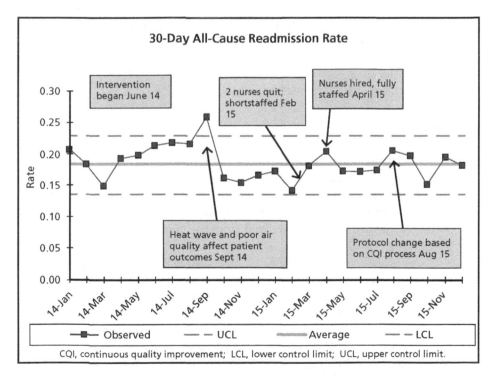

FIGURE 10.6   Noting important events on a control chart to better understand causes of variation.

BENCHMARKS

What Is Benchmarking?

Like SPC, benchmarking actually emerged from another field—industry. Robert Camp of Rank Xerox first realized that applying performance criteria to management techniques allowed for improved operation (Camp, 1989; McNair, 1992). Benchmarking has since morphed into a technique used in a large variety of fields and for many different purposes. In health care, benchmarking is most commonly utilized as part of CQI processes (Kay, 2007).

Whereas SPC methods can show whether or not the data are changing significantly over time, a limitation of these techniques is that they only measure outcomes against themselves in time. In other words, SPC can display whether or not a change has occurred in a process or outcome measure, but cannot show whether that measure is at an optimal level. In order to set goals and really understand the meaning of data, benchmarks are used as part of the data monitoring process to understand progress compared to best practices, to other similar populations, or to some other meaningful reference point.

Benchmarking is, at first glance, a process of establishing a standard from which to compare the program, processes, or outcomes in order to understand the relative meaning of the data. Benchmarking is generally considered to be part of a CQI process that shows how the procedures compare to best practices in order to improve health, efficiency, costs, quality, or satisfaction (McNair, 1992). Although, at its most basic, benchmarking is a method of identifying comparison points from which to understand the meaning of data, the nuances of benchmarking are in reality much more complex. There are many types of benchmarks that can be utilized, depending on the purpose and goals of a program or intervention. Whereas benchmarks are a very useful tool, they must be chosen very carefully in order to provide meaningful information.

Choosing a Benchmark

Selecting benchmarks should not be done in isolation; in fact, it is important to include the entire project team and leadership when determining what types of benchmarks to employ. Changing current practices may be necessary as part of a larger QI project, depending on how the data measure up to chosen benchmarks; therefore, having the team involved from the beginning to help select appropriate benchmarks is very essential.

As a team, it is important to take into account the purpose and goals set for the intervention. To understand how intervention goals affect the benchmark chosen, consider the following example. Suppose an intervention has been created to reduce readmissions for adults with chronic obstructive pulmonary disease (COPD). To understand the type of benchmark that would be appropriate for comparison, one must give thought to the goals of the program. Does the program have a goal of achieving the lowest rates of COPD readmissions among hospitals in the network? Is it focusing on hospitals with similar populations in the same state? Is it comparing outcomes to hospitals nationally? Is the goal to simply reduce COPD admissions to a standard level? Understanding the goals is the first step to selecting the type of benchmark to use.

Four main categories of benchmarks are:

- *Internal benchmarking*—Often internal benchmarking is done as a shared approach between departments in the same organization or organizations in the same network. It can also be done between populations who receive intervention and those who do not, in a comparison group-type approach (e.g., the team can compare an outcome of an intervention to a similar population at other hospitals who did not receive intervention). Internal benchmarking is usually a good way to establish a baseline performance level from which to monitor improvements or expand to external benchmarking efforts (McNair, 1992).
- *Competitive benchmarking*—Competitive benchmarking is often difficult because it relies on data sharing between competitors, such as two separately owned hospitals in the same region that wish to compare indicators for the purpose of QI. However, due to the accessibility of data made public online, in some instances competitive benchmarking can be done even when collaboration is not possible, although it will be limited by available data. Setting up QI partnerships between competitors can be a very valuable way to use benchmarks for mutual benefit; however, unless partnerships are already established, the amount of effort needed to do competitive benchmarking makes this option less appealing for many organizations (Kay, 2007; Pantall, 2001).
- *Functional benchmarking*—This type of benchmarking refers to comparative approaches to seeking best practices from similar fields or fields performing similar activities (e.g., comparing the registration of patients in a physician's office to checking in for airline passengers; Pantall, 2001). Functional benchmarking is less commonly used for clinical practice.
- *Generic benchmarking*—Generic benchmarking occurs between functions or processes that are the same but are taking place in different sectors (Kay, 2007). One instance would be a health care organization comparing its marketing strategy to the marketing strategy of a product retailer (Pantall, 2001).

For more information on each type of benchmark, see The Joint Commission's *Benchmarking in Health Care* (The Joint Commission Resources, 2011).

In clinical practice, it may be easiest to think of two categories of benchmarking: internal and external; that is, using data from within the health system—at the patient, practice, network, or health system levels—or at these same levels of external health systems—using data from other practices, other networks of practices, or national data. Benchmarks can be chosen to compare performance activities, patient experience, clinical outcomes, or quality measures from either internal or external sources (Kay, 2007).

Choosing Measures for Benchmarking

Once a team has a good understanding of the goals and the type of benchmarking that should be done, the type of process or activities to be benchmarked can be established. Ideally, benchmark choices should be considered early in the data management process—when developing process and outcome measures. The advantage to choosing benchmarks in tandem with measure development is that one can consider available benchmarks and the way they are described when developing measures for the intervention. The most relevant benchmarks are those that are calculated in the same way as the measures for an intervention. For example, if a team is gathering data on the number of readmissions among COPD patients and wants to use a benchmark to set goals for the program, the way a readmission is defined should be the same for both the program outcome and the benchmark. If the definition of a readmission is a second hospitalization within 60 days, for instance, and the benchmark defines a readmission as a second hospitalization within 90 days, it is very difficult to make a comparison between the figures.

Challenges in Benchmarking

Unfortunately, a serious challenge in benchmarking is finding comparable data to serve as a benchmark, especially when considering external benchmarks. Although internal benchmarking can offer the opportunity to create custom benchmarks from available data, external benchmarks are more often used to measure performance. Thus, limitations often exist due to lack of comparable data and measures. Following are important factors to consider when selecting an external benchmark.

TIMELINESS

One thing that makes benchmarking difficult is that benchmarks need to be regularly updated and timely to be relevant. In other words, it does not make much sense to use a disease benchmark from a decade ago to compare to the disease benchmark the team has chosen because so many contextual factors change over time. In order to be most useful, a benchmark should be recent and needs to be updated over time as the program is continuously monitored.

QUALITY OF BENCHMARK

The quality of the benchmark selected is also a key factor in the usefulness of the comparison. Utilizing a source of information that relies on a very small sample size, is drawn from an unreliable source, or relies on nonvalidated data sources and/or less rigorous methods for calculation should be done with caution.

COMPARABILITY

One of the biggest challenges in benchmarking is finding benchmarks that are comparable to the data collected. Ideal benchmarks come from a similar population with contextual factors similar to the one of interest. For example, comparing asthma rates in Medicaid children is most useful when an asthma benchmark is drawn from a population of children in Medicaid (not from a population of higher socioeconomic status, because socioeconomic factors often play a large role in asthma severity and therefore may be less comparable). Other factors to consider are contextual characteristics such as the type of facility from which data are drawn (e.g., a federally qualified health center or a private hospital), and the type of environment (urban or rural).

Internal benchmarking (and occasionally competitive benchmarking, when two entities work together to gather and share data) is the most likely to produce comparable data because teams define their own metrics and pull data that suit their needs. External benchmarks are often more limited for comparison purposes, because use of external benchmarks typically relies on existing indicators that are available, rather than forming partnerships among entities to gather data. In reality, it is very difficult to find benchmarks that are an exact comparison to the population of interest when the team relies on existing data sources; nevertheless, recognizing the limitations of the chosen benchmarks helps with interpretation of the comparison.

Sources of Health Care Benchmarks

As mentioned earlier, sources of health care benchmarks depend on the type of benchmarking process in place and the goals set for benchmarking as part of the ongoing monitoring process. If the team is using internal benchmarks or working externally with other organizations to collaboratively benchmark, data are usually drawn from these sources. However, if one plans to use publicly available benchmarks, there are many sources to explore. To illustrate, the Centers for Disease Control (CDC) website, healthdata.gov, the Dartmouth Atlas of Health Care, Agency for Healthcare Research and Quality (AHRQ), World Health Organization (WHO), Centers for Medicare and Medicaid Services (CMS), Data.gov.UK, and state health websites can all provide benchmarks for selected indicators. See Table 10.2 for examples of public data sources that can be used for benchmarking. In addition, many health organizations contract with consulting groups such as the Advisory Board Company, McKesson, or Milliman that can provide a wider range of benchmarks for more specific populations, although often with a cost attached.

Displaying Benchmark Data

Once benchmarking data have been gathered, these data should be displayed in a way most useful for ongoing monitoring. First, as discussed earlier, the team can display a benchmark in a column alongside the data gathered on the program in the form of a dashboard or table. Another more visual way to display benchmark data is to create an additional line that indicates the benchmark value on SPC charts or run charts. This allows a quick visual check of how program data compare with the benchmark selected. Figure 10.7 is an example of how a benchmark can be displayed on a control chart.

CONTINUOUS QUALITY IMPROVEMENT

CQI and Ongoing Monitoring

All ongoing monitoring activities are done for the same general purpose: to ensure that interventions are designed, implemented, and performed at the best level possible to maximize outcomes. However, although monitoring of process and outcome data through SPC and benchmarking can provide the information necessary to understand the processes and outcomes occurring after implementation,

TABLE 10.2 Sources for Data to Use for Benchmarking

Resources for Obtaining Public Benchmarks		
Organization	Types of Data	Website
Agency for Healthcare Research and Quality	Prevention Indicators, Health Care Disparities, Healthcare Cost and Utilization Project, HIV and AIDS Costs and Uses, Medical Expenditure Survey, Primary Care Workforce	http://www.ahrq.gov/research/data/dataresources.html
Centers for Disease Control and Prevention	Prevention Indicators, Community Health Status Indicators, Health Indicators Warehouse	http://www.cdc.gov/stltpublichealth/performance/data.html
Centers for Medicare and Medicaid Services (CMS)	Hospital Comparison Data, Medicaid Data, Nurse Home Comparison Data, Home Health Comparison Data	http://www.cms.gov
Dartmouth Atlas of Health Care	Care of Chronic Illness in Last Two Years of Life, Medicare Reimbursements, Hospital Use, Medical Discharges, Surgical Procedures, Post-Acute Care, Quality/Effectiveness of Care, Hospital and Physician Capacity, End of Life Care, Primary Care Service Area	http://www.dartmouthatlas.org
Data.Gov.UK	Health Behaviors; Accidents and Emergencies; Obesity, Diet, and Physical Activity Survey Data; Hospital Data; Dental Data	http://data.gov.uk/publisher/nhs-information-centre-for-health-and-social-care
Healthdata.gov	Medicare, Population Statistics, Administrative, Safety, Health Care Provider Data, Health Care Costs, Epidemiology, Biomedical Research, Medicaid, Quality Measurement, Treatments	http://healthdata.gov
The Joint Commission	Performance Measurement for Hospitals, Accountability Measures, Quality Check	http://www.jointcommission.org/performance_measurement.aspx
World Health Organization	Morbidity, Mortality, Diseases, Health System Indicators, Substance Abuse indicators, Millennium Development Goals	http://www.who.int/research/en/index.html

no positive changes can come about without incorporating all of these data into a larger CQI effort.

Like SPC and benchmarking, CQI methods arose from non–health care industries such as manufacturing that required constant monitoring of quality and rapid-cycle improvement processes to ensure and maintain a quality product (Kritchevsky & Simmons, 1991). Walter Shewhart and later W. E. Deming, among others, were responsible for translating QI theories into an organizational

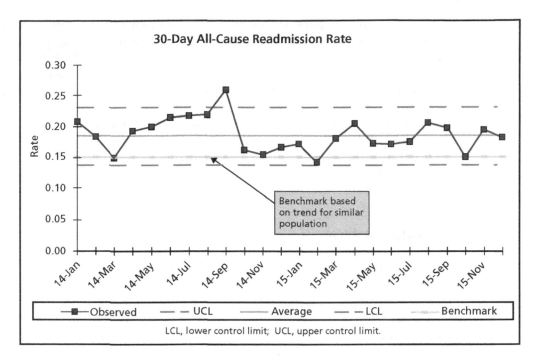

FIGURE 10.7   Displaying a benchmark on an SPC chart.

philosophy and management method (Kritchevsky & Simmons, 1991; Varkey, Reller, & Resar, 2007). CQI relies on the assumption that improving outcomes results from improving suboptimal processes, and this philosophy has been widely adopted across industries, including health care (Kritchevsky & Simmons, 1991; Radawski, 1999). There are various models for QI that may be adopted by organizations.

Types of CQI Models

CQI models typically follow the same pattern: understanding current practices, honing in on weak areas, and conducting rapid-cycle improvements for those processes that are weak in order to improve overall outcomes. Once a process has been modified, outcome measures that monitor the procedure improvements are used to make decisions on whether or not changes are effective. When changes are effective, the revisions should be maintained or expanded; when ineffective, process changes should be discontinued or modified. There are many QI models that can be used in health care settings, most of which follow this basic pattern. Following are a few examples of QI models used in health care:

1. *Plan–Do–Study–Act (PDSA)*—This model of QI is very popular and involves four steps: Plan, Do, Study, and Act. See Figure 10.8. This approach is focused on more in the next section (Institute for Healthcare Improvement, 2012; U.S. Department of Health and Human Services, n.d.).
2. *Focus, Analyze, Develop, Execute* (FADE)—This CQI model is similar to PDSA but involves the following steps: Focus, Analyze, Develop, Execute (U.S. Department of Health and Human Services, n.d).

■ *Six Sigma*—Another popular CQI model that originated from Motorola, Inc., in the 1980s is Six Sigma, an improvement system for existing processes that are not performing at an optimal level (Varkey et al., 2007). This model involves the following steps: define, measure, analyze, improve, control (Koning, Verver, Heuvel, Bisgaard, & Does, 2006; U.S. Department of Health and Human Services, n.d.).

■ *Lean Methodology*—Originally thought of as a process to reduce inefficiencies in procedures, this methodology relies on identifying the needs of the customer and improving processes through elimination of non–value-added activities (Varkey et al., 2007). This methodology helps create organization, clear work processes and standards, and efficiency in processes (Varkey et al., 2007).

One Example of a QI Method: PDSA

The PDSA model for QI is a staged approach to identifying weaknesses and addressing them (NHS Institute for Innovation and Improvement, 2008). This model relies directly on the ongoing monitoring outputs discussed in earlier sections, in order to conduct the first step: the Plan phase. Based on the data being monitored (and, in particular, on tools like SPC charts and benchmarking), the intervention team identifies weaknesses in project processes that are the focus of the first step in a CQI process.

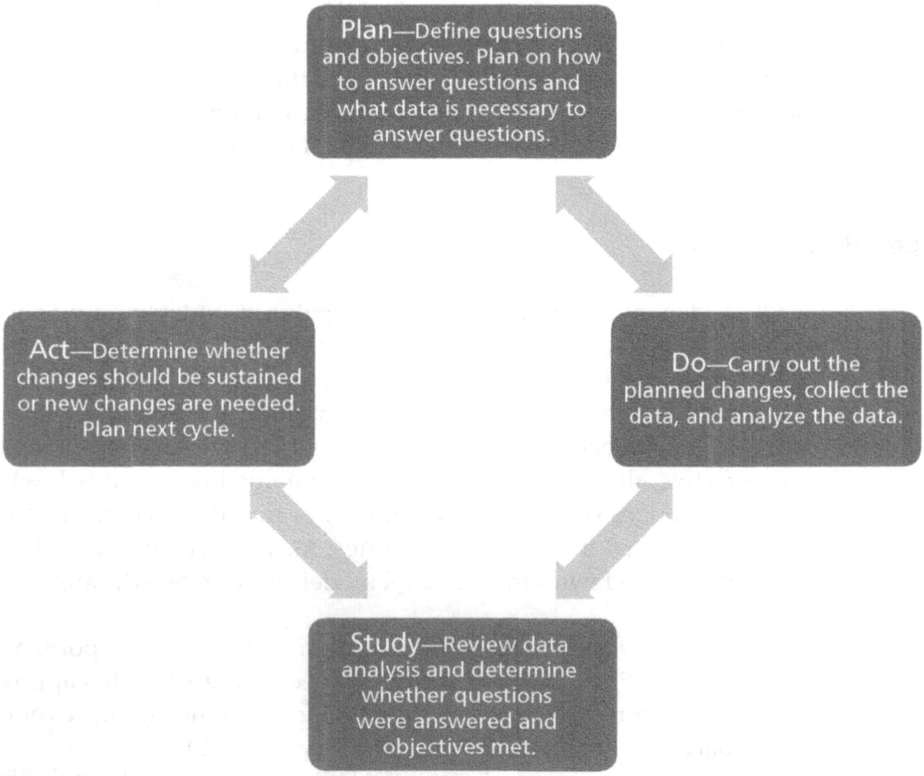

FIGURE 10.8 The PDSA cycle.
Adapted from NHS Institute for Innovation and Improvement (2008).

PLAN

Identifying opportunities for program improvement is the first step of the PDSA model: the "Plan" step. During the Plan step, the project team identifies a weakness, forms a new team of individuals who would best be able to understand and address the weakness identified, and plans for an improvement (NHS Institute for Innovation and Improvement, 2008). The team conducting QI may vary for each specific opportunity identified. For example, if an intervention is rolled out across various hospitals and overseen by a core oversight team, this team may identify a weakness in a process at an individual hospital that would be best understood and addressed by frontline workers at that site. The team conducting the Plan phase should assemble an improvement team carefully based on the process being studied, and everyone involved should have a clear role in the improvement process. The Plan phase is most effective when timelines and regular meetings are established to carry out improvements.

During the Plan phase, it is also important that team members have a clear aim that establishes what the group is trying to accomplish, how change is being measured, what success should look like, and what change should lead to that success. The change that is made should be based on a thorough analysis of the processes being addressed (NHS Institute for Innovation and Improvement, 2008). A fishbone diagram or other similar tool can help identify root causes for suboptimal results and can aid in identifying a solution. For more information on root cause analysis, see the U.S. Department of Veteran Affairs Root Cause Analysis website (U.S. Department of Veteran Affairs National Center for Patient Safety, 2007).

Ideally, by the end of the Plan phase, the team composition, the process needing improvement, the measure for success, the changes needed for improvement, and the goals of those changes should be established.

DO

In the next phase of this approach, the "Do" phase, the plan created for improvement of a process is carried out. After changes have been made, data are collected and displayed to understand whether the plan has been carried out successfully and whether or not changes have led to intended outcomes and improvements (NHS Institute for Innovation and Improvement, 2008). Run charts and control charts may be useful tools for understanding the results of the Do phase.

STUDY

Once changes have been established and data displayed, the "Study" phase of this cycle can be carried out. In this step, team members work together to understand the results of changes implemented, determine whether or not improvements have led to better processes or outcomes, and make a decision on whether or not the process has been successful (NHS Institute for Innovation and Improvement, 2008).

ACT

The "Act" phase comes about when the decision is made to retract changes (if the adjustments have been unsuccessful or have made a process worse), maintain revisions with new improvements (if there is still room for improvement in the process), or standardize the changes (if aims have been met and the process has been sufficiently improved to meet goals). At this point, once the cycle of PDSA has been completed, the decision can be made of whether to continue focusing on the problem originally identified, or to put other processes into PDSA cycles for improvement (NHS Institute for Innovation and Improvement, 2008). Cycles can be done for as many processes at a time as desired, assuming there are enough human resources to carry this out, and that the processes needing improvement are not all overlapping.

Each PDSA cycle addresses one specific area of opportunity for the intervention, and relies on strong monitoring data to be effective. Productive PDSA cycles require an engaged team with leadership buy-in to ensure that ongoing monitoring leads to QIs that can efficiently improve performance of an intervention. Implementing CQI cycles as part of an intervention offers the best opportunity to maximize outcomes of the intervention and iron out the process details that produce these outcomes. PDSA or other similar models offer the "what's next" step for patterns seen in data during the ongoing monitoring phase.

SUMMARY

Ongoing monitoring that is driven by program data is an essential step of any intervention. Whether data are displayed in a dashboard, graph, control chart, or other format, the way data are presented should vary by the needs and statistical knowledge of the audience. SPC charts and run charts are effective tools for monitoring program data for signs that a program is effective or ineffective in achieving its intended results (signs of special cause variation). Benchmarking provides a comparison of best practices or similar practices from which goals can be set and the performance of the program—both the processes and the outcomes—can be judged. These tools can be combined and then used as part of a CQI program that ensures the intervention is constantly improving in weak areas and is achieving the best possible outcomes.

REFERENCES

Benneyan, J., Lloyd, R., & Plsek, P. (2003). Statistical process control as a tool for research and healthcare improvement. *Quality and Safety in Health Care, 12*, 458–464.

Camp, R. (1989). *Benchmarking: The search for best industry practices that leads to superior performance.* Milwaukee, WI: ASQC Quality Press.

Carey, R. G. (2003). *Improving healthcare with control charts: Basic and advanced SPC methods and case studies.* Milwaukee, WI: ASQC Quality Press.

Institute for Healthcare Improvement. (2012, December 4). ihi.org. *How to improve.* Retrieved August 24, 2013, from http://www.ihi.org/knowledge/Pages/HowtoImprove/default.aspx

Kay, J. (2007). Health care benchmarking. *The Hong Kong Medical Diary, 12*(2), 22–27.

Koning, H., Verver, J., Heuvel, J., Bisgaard, S., & Does, R. (2006). Lean Six Sigma in healthcare. *Journal for Healthcare Quality, 28*(2), 4–11.

Kritchevsky, S., & Simmons, B. (1991). Continous quality improvement: Concepts and applications for physician care. *Journal of the American Medical Association, 266*(13), 1817–1823.

Marsteller, J., Huizinga, M., & Cooper, L. (2013). *Statistical process control: Possible uses to monitor and evaluate patient-centered medical home models.* Rockville, MD: Agency for Healthcare Research and Quality.

McNair, C. A. (1992). *Benchmarking: A tool for continuous improvement.* New York, NY: Harper Business.

NHS Institute for Innovation and Improvement. (2008). Quality and Service Improvement Tools. *Plan, do, study, act (PDSA).* Retrieved August 24, 2013, from http://www.institute.nhs.uk/quality_and_service_improvement_tools/quality_and_service_improvement_tools/plan_do_study_act.html

Pantall, J. (2001). Benchmarking in healthcare. *Journal of Research in Nursing, 6*(2), 568–580. 580–586.

Radawski, D. (1999). Continuous quality improvements: Origins, concepts, problems and applications. *Perspective on Physician Assistant Education, 10*(1), 12–16.

The Joint Commission Resources. (2011). *Benchmarking in health care.* Oak Brook, IL: Author.

Thor, J., Lundberg, J., Ask, J., Olsson, J., Carli, C., Harenstam, K., . . . Brommels, M. (2007). Application of statistical process control in healthcare improvement: Systematic review. *Quality and Safety in Health Care, 16*, 387–399.

U.S. Department of Health and Human Services. (n.d.). hrsa.gov. *What is quality improvement?* Retrieved August 24, 2013, from http://www.hrsa.gov/healthit/toolbox/HealthITAdoptiontoolbox/QualityImprovement/whatisqi.html

U.S. Department of Veteran Affairs National Center for Patient Safety. (2007). VA.gov. *Root cause analysis.* Retrieved 2013 from http://www.va.gov/NCPS/rca.html

Varkey, P., Reller, M., & Resar, R. (2007). Basics of quality improvement in health care. *Mayo Clinic Proceedings, 82*(6), 735–739.

CASE STUDY

CASE STUDY EXAMPLE: ONGOING MONITORING

SPC and Benchmarking

This case study focuses on one process measure (interventions have many processes occurring simultaneously; one example has been selected for the purposes of this case study) and three outcome measures: Rate of Admission, Rate of Readmissions, and Percentage of Patients with hemoglobin A1C (HbA1C) value in control (< 9%). Control charts in this section show each of the sigma lines in order to help determine significant changes in the data based on the tests noted in the SPC portion of this chapter.

PROCESS MEASURE

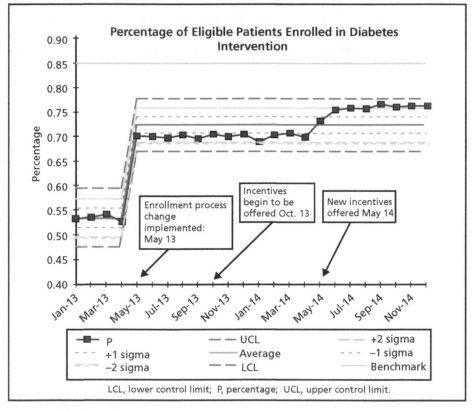

LCL, lower control limit; P, percentage; UCL, upper control limit.

- Enrollment rates started off well below the benchmark value of 85% enrollment among eligible patients. A PDSA cycle was initiated by a team to address this, and changes to the process were proposed.
- In April 2013, the changes to the enrollment process created by the continuous quality improvement (CQI) team resulted in a significant shift upward in the enrollment rates in May 2013.

- In October 2013, rates of enrollment were still not reaching the benchmark rate, so a CQI team again conducted a PDSA cycle. After root cause analysis, the team determined that incentives should be offered. The incentives did not create a significant change in the enrollment rates.
- A PDSA cycle was conducted again to reexamine incentive structure. New incentives were proposed and put into place on May 1, 2014. A significant upward trend in the data showed that new incentives significantly increased the enrollment rate among eligible patients. (Test 2: 2 of 3 successive points more than 2 sigma from the mean on the same side of the center line. Test 3: 4 out of 5 points more than 1 sigma from the mean on the same side of the center line. Test 4: 8 successive points on the same side of the center line.)

Outcome Measures

AVERAGE HbA1C

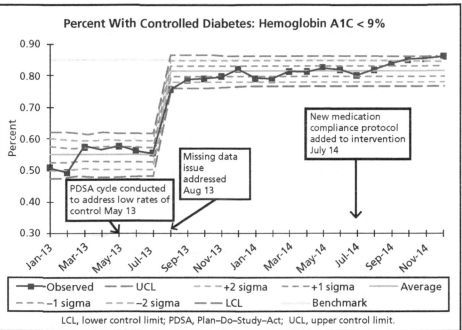

- HbA1C control rates remained low for the first quarter, with no significant changes to the data from January 2013 to June 2013. A PDSA cycle was conducted to address data issues around laboratory rates (see the following PDSA example).
- Significant shift in data took place in July 2013, after the PDSA cycle improved a data issue with lab values. This shift was due to a change in data, not a change in intervention.
- No significant shifts in diabetes control rates from August 2013 to July 2014.
- July 2014 through December 2014: Significant trend upward in percentage, with a controlled HbA1C value indicating that the medication compliance protocol may have succeeded in helping enrollees control their diabetes. (Test 2: 2 of 3 successive points more than 2 sigma from the mean on the same side of the center line. Test 5: 6 successive points increasing [a trend].)

ADMISSION RATE

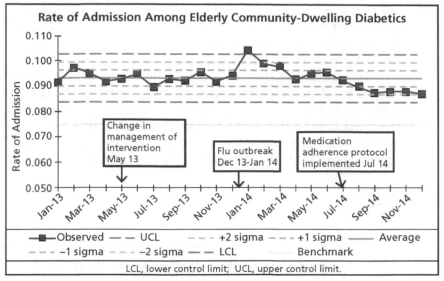

- No significant trends in data after change of management, and no other significant changes in rate of admission through the first 12 months of monitoring.
- In January 2014, a flu outbreak likely caused the significant increase in the number of admissions among intervention enrollees. (Test 1: 1 point outside the upper control limit.)
- It appears that the addition of the medication adherence protocol may have helped lower admission rates from July 2014 through December 2014. (Test 3: 4 out of 5 successive points more than 1 sigma from mean on same side of center line.)

READMISSION RATE

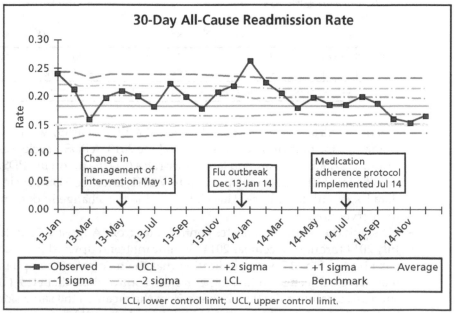

- The change in management did not appear to have a significant affect on the readmission rate for this intervention.
- Readmissions also significantly increased in January 2014, most likely due to the flu outbreak that caused an increase in the admission rate. (Test 1: 1 point outside the upper or lower control limits [UCLs, LCLs]. Test 2: 2 of 3 successive points more than 2 sigma from the mean on the same side of the center line.)
- No other significant trends appear in this chart, although several of the points do near the benchmark level of 15% of admissions resulting in readmission.

PDSA

To begin a PDSA cycle, the first step is to examine the data, such as the control charts shown for weaknesses in the program processes or outcomes. In these charts, a good example of how data changed based on efforts of the PDSA cycle can be seen in the HbA1C value control chart. Because interventions must be monitored from the beginning and PDSA cycles are ideally performed throughout the intervention, assume a team was formed to address the low rates of HbA1C control in this population in January 2013. By March 2013, it is clear that the rates of HbA1C control are much lower than the benchmark value, and therefore require attention. A team was formed to address this issue through a PDSA cycle. The following was the process that the team created:

Step 1: Plan

1. Look further into the data to try to understand if the low values are attributed to a measurement or data problem. If this is not the case and the data really represent poor HbA1C control among enrolled population, a root cause analysis should be performed to understand why enrollees have such poor HbA1C control, and what program aspects may need modification to improve rates of control.
2. The team discovers that laboratory values are not being reported from the vendor to the team in their entirety, and instead have a completion rate of only 54% for intervention enrollees who received the HbA1C test. All missing values are assumed to be out of control for the purposes of this measure, and because there is a high number of missing lab values, these then appear as out-of-control values in the measures and the true percentage of HbA1C control is difficult to determine. The team decides to take action on remedying the data reporting issue. The following represents their plan:

   - *Aim*: The team plans to improve the completion rates of lab values coming in from vendors in order to better understand diabetic control rates in the intervention population.
   - *Goal*: The team hopes that improving the completion rates of lab values reduces the number of enrollees with no known lab value and enables the team to better understand whether or not diabetes is well controlled in intervention enrollees. Having a clear understanding of the data should allow the team to better understand how far HbA1C control values are from the benchmark value so that further changes can be made if necessary.
   - *Measure of success*: 100% completion of lab data reporting with no missing values for enrollees who have received HbA1C tests.

▪ *Steps to execute*: Team to meet with each lab vendor to better understand why all lab values are not being reported. Team to work through a root cause analysis with lab vendors if a clear reason for missing values is not initially identified. Based on causes for missing data, team to determine if the lab vendors can solve the problem and report complete data, or if another source of data for labs is necessary to add. If lab vendors are unable to improve completion rates, team to work on linking electronic medical record data to intervention data in order to get lab data from another more complete source.

Step 2: Do

▪ In May 2013, team met with lab vendors to problem solve about why lab data being sent was incomplete. Lab vendors realized that there were issues with linkages between lab values and identification of intervention enrollees that were hindering completion of lab reporting. A plan was created to improve linkages through use of additional data and thereby increase completion rates of lab values.
▪ Lab vendors promised to fix linkage problem by July 2013.

Step 3: Study

▪ Team saw large increase in completion of lab data 2013 from 54% to 92% complete for the August 2013 reporting period.
▪ Based on the data and the SPC chart monitoring this measure, the team saw a large increase in the percentage of enrollees with controlled diabetes after lab data was improved. The SPC chart reflects this significant change in August 2013, at which point the team calculated a new mean and average to better monitor changes in values going forward. This gave the team a better sense of whether or not the intervention was helping control diabetes in enrollees since the data were more complete.

Step 4: Act

▪ The team continues to work with vendors to increase and maintain lab completion rates.
▪ The team reexamines the HbA1C control measure control chart on a monthly basis to better understand whether or not enrollees have controlled diabetes, or whether intervention processes need to be modified in order to best meet program goals of controlling diabetes to reduce admissions.

Index